The *Essential Clinical Skills for Nurses* series focuses on key clinical skills for nurses and other health professionals. These concise, accessible books assume no prior knowledge and focus on core clinical skills, clearly presenting common clinical procedures and their rationale, together with the essential background theory. Their user-friendly format makes them an indispensable guide to clinical practice for all nurses, especially to student nurses and newly qualified staff.

**Other titles in the *Essential Clinical Skills for Nurses* series:**

# Nursing Medical Emergency Patients

Edited by

## Philip Jevon
RN, BSc (Hons), PGCE, ENB 124
Resuscitation Officer/Clinical Skills Lead
Honorary Clinical Lecturer
Manor Hospital, Walsall, UK

## Melanie Humphreys
MA, BSc (Hons), DIPSIN, RGN, ONC, ENB 124
Senior Lecturer, Continuing Development Division
School of Health, University of Wolverhampton, UK

## Beverley Ewens
PG Dip Critical Care, BSc (Hons), PGCE, DPSN,
ENB 100, RGN
Staff Development Nurse, Practitioner Scholar
Joondalup Health Campus, Edith Cowan University
Western Australia

*Consulting Editors*
**Mr Saad Abdulla**
MBChB, DS, FRCS, DipMedTox, FCEM
Consultant in Emergency Medicine
Basildon University Hospital, UK

**Adam Crawford McGuffie**
MBChB, MRCP, FCEM
Consultant in Emergency Medicine
Emergency Department
Crosshouse Hospital, Ayrshire, UK

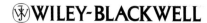

## WILEY-BLACKWELL

A John Wiley & Sons, Ltd., Publication

This edition first published 2008
© 2008 Blackwell Publishing Ltd

Blackwell Publishing was acquired by John Wiley & Sons in February 2007.
Blackwell's publishing programme has been merged with Wiley's global
Scientific, Technical, and Medical business to form Wiley-Blackwell.

*Registered office*
John Wiley & Sons Ltd, The Atrium, Southern Gate, Chichester, West
Sussex, PO19 8SQ, United Kingdom

*Editorial offices*
9600 Garsington Road, Oxford, OX4 2DQ, United Kingdom
350 Main Street, Malden, MA 02148-5020, USA

For details of our global editorial offices, for customer services and for information about how to apply for permission to reuse the copyright material in
this book please see our website at www.wiley.com/wiley-blackwell.

*Library of Congress Cataloging-in-Publication Data*

Jevon, Philip.
Nursing medical emergency patients / Philip Jevon, Beverley Ewens,
Melanie Humphreys.
p. ; cm. – (Essential clinical skills for nurses)
Includes bibliographical references and index.
ISBN 978-1-4051-2055-5 (pbk. : alk. paper)  1. Emergency
nursing.  I. Ewens, Beverley.  II. Humphreys,
Melanie.  III. Title.  IV. Series.
[DNLM:  1. Emergencies–nursing.  2. Critical Care–
methods.  3. Nursing Care–methods. WY 154 J58n 2008]
RT120.E4J49 2008
610.73′6–dc22
2007047498

A catalogue record for this book is available from the British Library.

Set in 9 on 12 pt Palatino by SNP Best-set Typesetter Ltd., Hong Kong
Printed and bound in Malaysia by Vivar Printing Sdn Bhd.

1  2008

# Contents

# Contributors

**Anthony Batson** RMN, RGN, ENB 100, ENB 148, DN (LON), RCNT, RNT, BSc (Hons)
Senior Lecturer, Pre-registration Studies, University of Wolverhampton, Wolverhampton, UK

**James Bethel** RN, Emergency Nurse Practitioner, BSc (Hons) Clinical practice, PGD Emergency Care, PGC Learning and Teaching in HE
Senior Lecturer, Emergency Medicine, University of Wolverhampton, Wolverhampton, UK

**Kate Deacon** PgDip (Health Psychology), BA (Hons) Psychology, RGN, ENB 100
Senior Lecturer, Intensive Care, University of Wolverhampton, Wolverhampton, UK

**Beverley Ewens,** PG Dip Critical Care, BSc (Hons), PGCE, DPSN, ENB 100, RGN
Staff Development Nurse Practitioner Scholar, Joondalup Health Campus, Edith Cowan University, Western Australia

**Fiona Foxall** MA Medical Ethics & Law, BSc (Hons) Nursing Studies, DPSN, PGCE (FAHE), ENB 100, RGN
Head of Division, Continuing Professional Development, University of Wolverhampton, Wolverhampton, UK

**Melanie Humphreys** MA, BSc (Hons), DIPSIN, RGN, ONC, ENB 124
Senior Lecturer, Continuing Development Division, School of Health, University of Wolverhampton, Wolverhampton, UK

**Philip Jevon** RN, BSc (Hons), PGCE, ENB 124
Resuscitation Officer/Clinical Skills Lead, Honorary Clinical
  Lecturer, Manor Hospital, Walsall, UK

**Gillian Maidens** RMN, BSc (Hons), PGCE (Cert. ed)
  Senior Lecturer, Mental Health, University of
  Wolverhampton, Wolverhampton, UK

**Sue Talbot** MSc Advanced Nursing Practice, BSc (Hons)
  Educational Studies (Nursing), ENB 136, RNT, RGN
Senior Lecturer, Renal Care, University of Wolverhampton,
  Wolverhampton, UK

**Christine Thompson** PGDE, BSc, ENB 199, RGN
Senior Lecturer, Pre-registration Studies, University of
  Wolverhampton, Wolverhampton, UK

# Foreword

Historically in the UK, medical emergencies would have occurred within limited areas within the acute hospital such as the emergency department, theatres and recovery and critical care units. However, a number of factors such as a shift of emphasis to care in the community, reduced hospital bed capacity and advanced medical technologies have resulted in hospital beds being occupied by only the acutely ill. This has necessitated all nurses working within the in-patient environment needing to recognise medical emergencies promptly and to instigate appropriate resuscitation. Delay in recognising signs and symptoms of deteriorating medical status can be fatal or severely compromise the patient's full recovery to health. Furthermore, with the government directives to reduce junior doctors' working hours nurses are in a pivotal position to be first responders to medical emergencies. Demographically, the UK has an ageing population and this has led to a dramatic increase in the number of people with several co-morbid long terms conditions such as heart failure, chronic respiratory and renal disease. Thus, even patients admitted to hospital for fairly routine procedures or investigations are likely to be predisposed to developing complications such as cardiac failure, pulmonary embolism and shock.

This text provides a user friendly and practical aid to student nurses and registered nurses who wish to further develop their knowledge and skills in responding to medical emergencies effectively. The text does not require the reader to have any previous experience of caring for emergency medical patients as it provides clear and precise guidance to all stages of the ABCDE approach for the most frequently occurring medical emergency situations. Chapter 12 assists us to understand the many complex ethical and legal issues related to the care and treatment of emergency patients in contemporary health care. The editors and contributors are to be commended on compiling this extremely useful text, which should be on the essential reading list for all pre-registration nursing curricula. In summary, this text emphasises the importance of thorough patient observation, which was recognised by Florence Nightingale who wrote

'In dwelling upon the vital importance of observation, it must never be lost sight of what observation is for. It is not for the sake of piling up miscellaneous information or curious facts, but for the sake of saving life and increasing health and comfort' (Nightingale, 1859)

### REFERENCE

Nightingale, F (1859) *Notes on Nursing.* J B Lippincott, Philadelphia.

# Acknowledgements

We extend our thanks to the contributing authors for their valuable contribution to this book. We have relied on their appraisal of the current literature, national recommendations e.g. Resuscitation Council (UK), National Institute for Clinical Excellence (NICE) and local guidelines, policies and procedures, together with utilising their clinical experience and expertise.

We are particularly grateful to our two Consulting Editors, Dr Adam Crawford McGuffie and Mr Saad Abdulla, for kindly reviewing the clinical accuracy of the text and making helpful and valuable suggestions to improve it.

Finally we are grateful to the staff at Blackwell Publishing for their advice, continued support and patience in all aspects of the publishing process.

Philip Jevon
Melanie Humphreys
Beverley Ewens

# Overview of the Treatment of Medical Emergencies

**1**

## Philip Jevon

## INTRODUCTION

Medical emergencies can be life-threatening. Prompt recognition and effective early treatment of a patient with a medical emergency is paramount if deterioration of the patient is to be prevented and the chances of recovery are to be maximised. The aim of this book is to understand the treatment of medical emergencies.

The assessment and treatment of any patient with a medical emergency should follow the ABCDE approach advocated by the Resuscitation Council UK (Resuscitation Council UK, 2006). In this chapter a brief overview to this generic approach will be provided (a more detailed and comprehensive guide can be found in *Treating the Critically Ill Patient*, Jevon, 2007) and throughout the book its importance will be continually emphasised.

The aim of this chapter is to provide an overview to the treatment of medical emergencies.

## LEARNING OUTCOMES

At the end of the chapter the reader will be able to:

❏ list what emergency equipment should be available,
❏ describe the assessment of a patient with a medical emergency,
❏ state the aim of treating a patient with a medical emergency.

This chapter is based on the chapter 'Overview of Treating the Critically Ill Patient' which first appeared in *Treating the Critically Ill Patient* by Jevon (2007). It has been revised and updated.

## EMERGENCY EQUIPMENT

Wherever patients with medical emergencies are treated, procedures should be in place to ensure that all the essential monitoring and emergency equipment and emergency drugs/fluids are immediately available, accessible and in good working order (Jevon, 2001).

### Oxygen

Facilities should be available for the delivery of high concentrations of oxygen: either piped oxygen to a wall-outlet behind the patient's bed (preferable), or a portable oxygen cylinder, fitted with a variable oxygen-flow-rate meter capable of delivering up to 15 litres/min (Figure 1.1). There should also be adequate stocks of various oxygen-delivery devices, particularly non-rebreathe masks (see Figure 1.4, below).

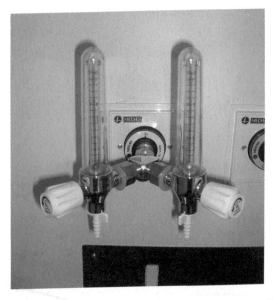

**Figure 1.1** A wall mounted oxygen cylinder, fitted with a variable oxygen-flow-rate meter capable of delivering up to 15 litres/min

## Suction

Every clinical area should have access to a portable suction device. In addition, it is preferable if a wall-mounted suction device is available behind each patient's bed (Figure 1.2). As suction is sometimes required immediately in a life-threatening situation, it is standard practice to store appropriate suction connection tubing, together with suction catheters (rigid and flexible), with the suction source; that is, suction can be quickly administered.

## Monitoring devices

At the very least, an ECG monitor and a pulse oximeter should be available. Other monitoring facilities, for example capnography, may also be required in some clinical areas.

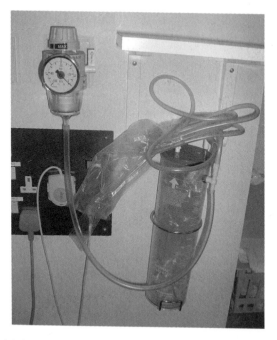

**Figure 1.2** A wall-mounted suction device

## Cardiopulmonary resuscitation trolley

A carefully set out and fully stocked cardiac arrest trolley is paramount, following Resuscitation Council guidelines (Box 1.1) (Resuscitation Council UK, 2004). The trolley should be spacious, sturdy, easily accessible and mobile; ideally each trolley in a healthcare establishment should be identically stocked to avoid confusion. A defibrillator should be immediately available and, where

---

### Box 1.1 Cardiopulmonary resuscitation equipment that should be available

#### Airway equipment

- Pocket mask with oxygen port (should be widely available in all clinical areas)
- Self-inflating resuscitation bag with oxygen reservoir and tubing (ideally, the resuscitation bag should be single-use; if not, it should be equipped with a suitable filter)
- Clear face masks, sizes 3, 4 and 5
- Oropharyngeal airways, sizes 2, 3 and 4
- Nasopharyngeal airways, sizes 6 and 7
- Portable suction equipment
- Yankauer suckers
- Tracheal suction catheters, sizes 12 and 14
- Laryngeal mask airways (LMAs; sizes 4 and 5), or ProSeal LMAs (sizes 4 and 5), or Combitube (small)
- Magill forceps
- Tracheal tubes, oral, cuffed, sizes 6, 7 and 8
- Gum elastic bougie or equivalent device
- Lubricating jelly
- Laryngoscope handles (×2) and blades (standard and long blade)
- Spare batteries for laryngoscope and spare bulbs (if applicable)
- Fixation for tracheal tube (e.g. ribbon gauze/tape)
- Scissors
- Selection of syringes
- Oxygen mask with reservoir (non-rebreathing) bag
- Oxygen cylinders
- Cylinder key

---

**Circulation equipment**

- Defibrillator (shock advisory module and or external pacing facility to be decided by local policy)
- ECG electrodes
- Defibrillation gel pads or self-adhesive defibrillator pads (preferred)
- Selection of intravenous cannulae
- Selection of syringes and needles
- Cannula fixing dressings and tapes
- Seldinger central venous catheter kit
- Intravenous infusion sets
- 0.9% sodium chloride, 1000 ml × 2
- Arterial blood gas syringes
- Tourniquet

**Drugs**

(a) Immediately available prefilled syringes
- Adrenaline (epinephrine) 1 mg (1:10,000) × 4
- Atropine 3 mg × 1
- Amiodarone 300 mg × 1
(b) Other readily available drugs

*IV injections*

- Adenosine 6 mg × 10
- Adrenaline 1 mg (1:10,000) × 4
- Adrenaline 1 mg (1:1000) × 2
- Amiodarone 300 mg × 1
- Calcium chloride 10 ml of 100 mg/ml × 1
- Chlorphaniramine 10 mg × 2
- Furosemide 50 mg × 2
- Glucose 10% 500 ml × 1
- Hydrocortisone 100 mg × 2
- Lignocaine 100 mg
- Magnesium sulphate 50% solution 2 g (4 ml) × 1
- Midazolam 10 mg × 1
- Naloxone 400 μg × 5
- Normal saline, 10 ml ampoules
- Potassium chloride for injection (see National Patient Safety Agency Alert, www.npsa.nhs.uk)

*Continued*

- Sodium bicarbonate 8.4%, 50 ml × 1

*Other medications/equipment*
- Salbutamol (5 mg × 2) and ipratropium bromide (500 µg × 2) nebules
- Nebulizer device and mask
- Glyceryl trinitrate spray
- Aspirin 300 mg

**Additional items**
- Clock
- Gloves/goggles/aprons
- Audit forms
- Sharps container and clinical waste bag
- Large scissors
- Alcohol wipes
- Blood sample bottles
- A sliding sheet or similar device should be available for safer handling

Source: Resuscitation Council UK (2004).

appropriate, for example on general wards, it should have an automatic or advisory facility (Jevon, 2001). Defibrillators with external pacing should be strategically located, for example in emergency departments, intensive care units (ICUs) and coronary care units (CCUs).

**Routine checking of emergency equipment**
All emergency equipment should be checked routinely following local protocols. It is recommended that cardiopulmonary resuscitation equipment should be checked on a daily basis by each ward or department responsible for it (Resuscitation Council UK, 2000). A system for daily documented checks of the equipment inventory should be in place (Jevon, 2001). The electronic equipment should be stored, maintained and checked following the manufacturer's recommendations and those of the local electrobiomedical engineers' department (EBME).

## ASSESSMENT OF A PATIENT WITH A MEDICAL EMERGENCY

### ABCDE assessment

A patient with a medical emergency will be critically ill. The Resuscitation Council UK (2006) has issued guidelines on the recognition and treatment of the critically ill patient. Adapted from the ALERT course (Smith, 2003), these guidelines follow the logical and systematic ABCDE approach to patient assessment and treatment:

- **A**irway,
- **B**reathing,
- **C**irculation,
- **D**isability,
- **E**xposure.

When assessing the patient, a complete initial assessment should be undertaken, identifying and treating life-threatening problems first, before moving on to the next part of assessment. The effectiveness of treatment/intervention should be evaluated, and regular re-assessment undertaken. The need to alert more senior help should be recognised and other members of the multidisciplinary team should be utilised as appropriate so that patient assessment, instigation of appropriate monitoring and interventions can be undertaken simultaneously.

Irrespective of their training, experience and expertise in clinical assessment and treatment, all nurses can follow the ABCDE approach; clinical skills, knowledge, expertise and local circumstances will determine what aspects of the assessment and treatment are undertaken. Throughout this book, the ABCDE approach will be reinforced.

### Prevention of cross-infection

When assessing and treating the critically ill patient, it is important to ensure that effective measures are taken to minimise the

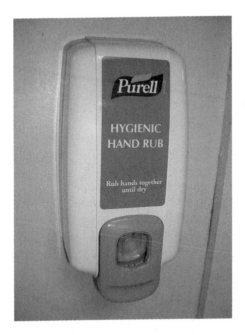

**Figure 1.3** Hygienic hand-rub

risk of cross-infection. Wash hands or use alcohol gel following local policy (Figure 1.3).

### Communication with the patient

Talk to the patient and evaluate the response: a normal response indicates that they have a clear airway, are breathing and have adequate cerebral perfusion; if they are unable to complete sentences in one breath, this may be an indication of extreme respiratory distress. An inappropriate response or no response could indicate an acute life-threatening physiological disturbance (Gwinnutt, 2006).

### General appearance of the patient

Note the patient's general appearance, their colour and whether they appear content and relaxed or distressed and anxious.

## Senior help

During the assessment process, consider whether senior help should be requested. Evaluate MEWS score and alert medics/outreach if necessary (see p. 298).

## Oxygen

Administer high concentrations of oxygen: use a non-rebreathe mask (Figure 1.4) connected to an oxygen flow rate of 15 litres/min (Smith, 2003). This will enable the delivery of an inspired oxygen concentration of approximately 95% (Jevon, 2007). Prior to application, carry out checks to ensure correct functioning as recommended by the manufacturer (Figure 1.5).

## Patient-monitoring devices

Attach appropriate monitoring devices, for example pulse oximetry, ECG monitor and non-invasive blood-pressure

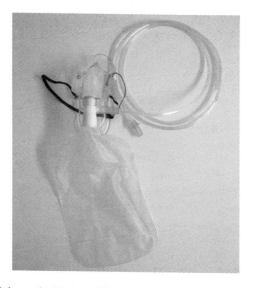

**Figure 1.4** A non-rebreathe mask. Taken from Jevon, P (2007) *Treating the Critically Ill Patient*. Blackwell Publishing, Oxford, with permission

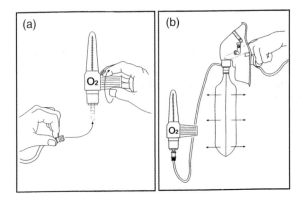

**Figure 1.5** Ensure correct functioning as recommended by the manufacturer. (a) Attach the tubing to the oxygen source and set the oxygen flow rate. (b) Occlude the valve between the mask and the oxygen reservoir bag to check that the bag fills up with oxygen. Taken from Jevon, P (2007) *Treating the Critically Ill Patient.* Blackwell Publishing, Oxford, with permission.

monitoring, as soon as it is safe to do so (Resuscitation Council UK, 2006).

**Assessment of airway**

Look, listen and feel for the signs of airway obstruction. Partial airway obstruction will result in noisy breathing:

- *gurgling*: indicates the presence of fluid, for example secretions or vomit, in the mouth or upper airway; usually seen in a patient with altered conscious level who is having difficulty or is unable to clear their own airway;
- *snoring*: indicates that the pharynx is being partially obstructed by the tongue; usually seen in a patient with altered conscious level lying in a supine position;
- *stridor*: high-pitched sound during inspiration, indicating partial upper-airway obstruction; usually due to either a foreign body or laryngeal oedema;
- *wheeze*: noisy musical whistling type sound due to the turbulent flow of air through narrowed bronchi and bronchioles,

more pronounced on expiration; causes include asthma and chronic obstructive pulmonary disease (COPD).

Complete airway obstruction can be detected by no air movement at the patient's mouth and nose. Paradoxical chest and abdominal movements ('see-saw' movement of the chest) may be observed; central cyanosis (a late sign of airway obstruction) will develop if not treated rapidly.

If the patient's airway is compromised, or is at risk of being compromised, take immediate action. Treat the underlying cause (Resuscitation Council UK, 2006); for example:

- apply head tilt/chin lift to open the airway;
- suction the airway if secretions, blood or gastric contents are present;
- place the patient in the lateral position if breathing, but has altered conscious level;
- if the patient is unconscious, insert an oropharyngeal airway to help maintain an oral airway (a nasopharyngeal airway may be helpful in a patient who is semi-conscious);
- advanced airway intervention, for example tracheal intubation or tracheostomy, may be required in some situations;
- administer high-concentration oxygen.

### Assessment of breathing

Look, listen and feel to assess breathing.

*Count the respiratory rate:* normal respiratory rate is 12–20 breaths/ min (Resuscitation Council UK, 2006). Tachypnoea is usually the first sign that the patient has a physiological upset, the cause of which may be respiratory (NCEPOD, 2005). Bradypnoea is an ominous sign and could indicate imminent respiratory arrest; causes include drugs such as opiates, fatigue, hypothermia, head injury and central nervous system depression.

*Evaluate chest movement:* chest movement should be symmetrical; unilateral chest movement suggests unilateral pathology, such as pneumothorax, pneumonia or pleural effusion (Smith, 2003).

*Evaluate depth of breathing:* only marked degrees of hyperventilation and hypoventilation can be detected; hyperventilation may be seen in metabolic acidosis or anxiety and hypoventilation may be seen in opiate toxicity (Ford et al., 2005).

*Evaluate respiratory pattern:* a Cheyne–Stokes breathing pattern (periods of apnoea alternating with periods of hyperpnoea) can be associated with brain-stem ischaemia, cerebral injury and severe left-ventricular failure (altered carbon dioxide sensitivity of the respiratory centre) (Ford et al., 2005).

*Note the oxygen saturation (SpO₂) reading:* 97–100% is normal. A low $SpO_2$ could indicate respiratory distress or compromise. Note that the pulse oximeter does not detect hypercapnia and that the $SpO_2$ can be normal in the presence of a very high $PaCO_2$ (Resuscitation Council UK, 2006).

*Listen to the breathing:* normal breathing is quiet. Rattling airway noises indicate the presence of airway secretions, usually due to the patient being unable to cough sufficiently or unable to take a deep breath in (Smith, 2003). The presence of stridor or wheeze indicates partial, but significant, airway obstruction (see above).

*Check the position of the trachea:* place the tip of the index finger into the suprasternal notch, let it slip either side of the trachea and determine whether it fits more easily into one or other side of the trachea (Ford et al., 2005). Deviation of the trachea to one side indicates mediastinal shift (e.g. lung collapse, pneumothorax, lung fibrosis or pleural fluid).

*Palpate the chest wall:* to detect surgical emphysema or crepitus (suggesting a pneumothorax *until* proven otherwise) (Smith, 2003).

*Perform chest percussion:* this is done as follows.

- Place the left hand on the patient's chest wall. Ensure that the fingers are separated slightly, with the middle finger pressed firmly into the intercostal space to be percussed (Ford et al., 2005).

- Strike the centre of the middle phalanx of the middle finger sharply using the tip of the middle finger of the right hand (Ford et al., 2005). Deliver the stroke using a quick flick of the wrist and finger joints not from the arm or shoulder. The percussing finger should be bent so that its terminal phalanx is at right angles to the metacarpal bones when the blow is delivered, and it strikes the percussed finger in a perpendicular way. The percussing finger should then be removed immediately, like a clapper inside a bell, otherwise the resultant sound will be dampened (Epstein et al., 2003).
- Percuss the anterior and lateral chest wall. Percuss from side to side, top to bottom, comparing both sides and looking for asymmetry.
- Categorise the percussion sounds (see below).
- If an area of altered resonance is located, map out its boundaries by percussing from areas of normal to altered resonance (Ford et al., 2005).
- Sit the patient forward and then percuss the posterior chest wall, omitting the areas covered by the scapulae. Ask the patient to move their elbows forward across the front of the chest: this will rotate the scapulae anteriorly and out of the way (Talley & O'Connor, 2001). It may be helpful to offer the patient a pillow to lean on.
- Again percuss from side to side, top to bottom, comparing both sides and looking for asymmetry. Don't forget that the lung extends much further down posteriorly than anteriorly (Epstein et al., 2003).
- Categorise the percussion sounds (see below).

The causes of different percussion notes are listed below (source, Ford et al., 2005):

- *resonant*: air-filled lung;
- *dull*: liver, spleen, heart, lung consolidation/collapse;
- *stony dull*: pleural effusion/thickening;
- *hyper-resonant*: pneumothorax, emphysema;
- *tympanitic*: gas-filled viscus.

### Auscultate the chest

- Ask the patient to breathe in and out normally through their mouth.
- Auscultate the anterior chest from side to side, and top to bottom. Auscultate over equivalent areas and compare the volume and character of the sounds and note any additional sounds. Compare the sounds during inspiration and expiration.
- Note the location and quality of the sounds heard.
- Auscultate the posterior chest, from side to side, and top to bottom. Auscultate over equivalent areas and compare the volume and character of the sounds and note any additional sounds. Compare the sounds during inspiration and expiration (Jevon & Cunnington, 2006).

Evaluate air entry, the depth of breathing and the equality of breath sounds on both sides of the chest. Bronchial breathing indicates lung consolidation; absent or reduced sounds suggest a pneumothorax or pleural fluid (Smith, 2003). In particular, note any additional breath sounds:

- *Wheezes (rhonchi)*: these are high-pitched musical sounds associated with air being forced through narrowed airways, for example asthma (Ford et al., 2005). This is usually more pronounced on expiration. Inspiratory wheeze (stridor) is usually indicative of severe upper-airway obstruction, for example by a foreign body or laryngeal oedema. If both inspiratory and expiratory wheezes are heard, this is usually due to excessive airway secretions (Adam & Osborne, 2005).
- *Crackles (crepitations)*: these are non-musical sounds, associated with reopening of a collapsed airway, for example pulmonary oedema (Ford et al., 2005). Crackles are usually localised in pneumonia and mild cases of bronchiectasis; in pulmonary oedema and fibrosing alveolitis, both lung bases are affected equally (Epstein et al., 2003).
- *Pleural friction rub*: this can be heard as leathery/creaking sounds during inspiration and expiration, evident in areas

of inflammation when the normally smooth pleural surfaces are roughened and rub on each other (Adam & Osborne, 2005).

*Record peak expiratory flow rate:* this provides a useful estimate of the calibre of the airways, particularly in asthma and COPD (Ford et al., 2005).

### Evaluate the efficacy of breathing, work of breathing and adequacy of ventilation

- *Efficacy of breathing*: air entry, chest movement, pulse oximetry, arterial blood gas analysis and capnography.
- *Work of breathing*: respiratory rate and use of accessory muscles, for example neck and abdominal muscles.
- *Adequacy of ventilation*: heart rate, skin colour and mental status.

If breathing is compromised, ensure a clear airway and administer a high concentration of oxygen. Positioning the patient in an upright position can be helpful in a patient who is breathing spontaneously. It is important to recognise and effectively treat immediately life-threatening conditions, such as acute severe asthma, pulmonary oedema, tension pneumothorax and massive haemothorax (Resuscitation Council UK, 2006). Patients with inadequate ventilation will need ventilatory support.

### Assessment of circulation

Look, listen and feel to assess circulation.

*Palpate peripheral and central pulses:* check for presence, rate, quality, regularity and equality (Smith, 2003). A weak, thready pulse suggests a poor cardiac output and a bounding pulse may indicate sepsis (Resuscitation Council UK, 2006).

*Check the colour and temperature of the hands and fingers:* signs of cardiovascular compromise include cool and pale peripheries.

*Measure the capillary refill time (CRT):* apply sufficient pressure to cause blanching to the skin, for example on the sternum, for 5 s and then release (Figure 1.6). Normal CRT is less than 2 s; a

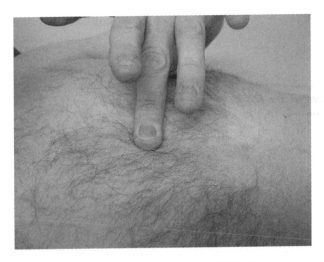

**Figure 1.6** Measuring the central capillary refill time (CRT). Taken from Jevon, P (2007) *Treating the Critically Ill Patient.* Blackwell Publishing, Oxford, with permission

prolonged CRT could indicate poor peripheral perfusion, although other causes can include cool ambient temperature, poor lighting and old age (Resuscitation Council UK, 2006).

*Look for other signs of a poor cardiac output:* these include altered conscious level and, if the patient has a urinary catheter, oliguria (urine volume less than 0.5 ml/kg per h) (Smith, 2003).

*Look for signs of haemorrhage:* for example from wounds or drains, or evidence of internal haemorrhage, such as abdominal swelling; concealed blood loss can be significant, even if drains are empty (Smith, 2003).

*Measure blood pressure:* systolic blood pressure (BP) of less than 90 mmHg suggests shock. A normal BP does not exclude shock because compensatory mechanisms increase peripheral resistance in response to reduced cardiac output (Smith, 2003). A low diastolic BP suggests arterial vasodilatation, for example anaphylaxis or sepsis. A narrowed pulse pressure – that is, the difference between systolic and diastolic readings (normal is

35–45 mmHg), suggests arterial vasoconstriction, for example cardiogenic shock or hypovolaemia (Resuscitation Council UK, 2006).

*Assess the state of the veins:* if hypovolaemia is present the veins could be under-filled or collapsed (Smith, 2003).

*Interpret the ECG:* determine whether a cardiac arrhythmia is present. A 12-lead ECG should be recorded as a priority in some situations, for example chest pain.

If the patient has compromised circulation (Resuscitation Council UK, 2006);

- ensure the airway is clear and breathing is adequate;
- administer high-concentration oxygen;
- if shock present, insert one or more wide-bore cannulae (14–16-gauge), and start treatment directed at fluid replacement, haemorrhage control and restoration of tissue perfusion; administer a rapid fluid challenge, for example 500 ml normal saline (warmed) over 5–10–min;
- if the patient has chest pain and acute coronary syndrome is suspected, treat initially with oxygen, aspirin, nitroglycerine and morphine.

### Assessment of disability

Assess disability (central nervous system function) as follows.

*Evaluate the patient's level of consciousness:* use the AVPU scale (see Box 6.1) or the Glasgow Coma Scale (GCS) (see Box 6.2) if a more objective assessment of conscious level is required, for example head injury (see Chapter 6 in this volume).

*Examine the pupils:* compare size, equality and reaction to light of each pupil.

*Undertake bedside glucose measurement:* exclude hypoglycaemia as a cause of altered conscious level.

If the patient has altered conscious level (Resuscitation Council UK, 2006):

- review ABC: exclude or treat hypoxia and hypotension (both of which are possible causes of altered conscious level);
- nurse in a lateral position, with particular attention to the airway;
- review the patient's medication chart: check for reversible medication-induced causes of altered conscious level, for example administer naloxone (opioid antagonist) for opioid toxicity.

### Exposure

Expose the patient and undertake a thorough examination to ensure that important details are not over-looked (Smith, 2003). In particular, the examination should concentrate on the part of the body that is most probably contributing to the patient's ill status, for example in suspected anaphylaxis, examine the skin for urticaria. Respect the patient's dignity and minimise heat loss.

In addition (source, Resuscitation Council UK, 2006):

- take a full clinical history and review the patient's notes/charts;
- study the recorded vital signs: trends are more significant than one-off recordings;
- administer prescribed medications;
- review laboratory results and ECG and radiological investigations;
- ascertain what level of care the patient requires (e.g. ward, high-dependency unit, ICU);
- document in the patient's notes details of assessment, treatment and response to treatment.

### THE AIM OF TREATING A PATIENT WITH A MEDICAL EMERGENCY

The aim of treating a patient with a medical emergency is the early anticipation and detection of abnormal physiology at a stage before organ failure is established and to initiate simple preventative therapies and interventions (Smith, 2003). The initial ABCDE assessment and treatment should be seen as a holding measure to keep the patient alive, and to produce some clinical improvement, so that definitive treatment may be initiated (Resuscitation Council UK, 2006). The aim of this book is to discuss the treatment of medical emergencies following the ABCDE approach.

## CONCLUSION

Recognition and the effective treatment of a patient with a medical emergency is paramount. In this chapter the importance of ensuring that the necessary emergency equipment is available and the systematic approach to assessment following the ABCDE method have been described. In the remaining chapters of the book the specific treatment for individual medical emergencies will be discussed.

## REFERENCES

Adam, S & Osborne, S (2005) *Critical Care Nursing Science and Practice*, 2nd edn. Oxford University Press, Oxford

Epstein, O, Perkin, G, Cookson, J & de Bono, D (2003) *Clinical Examination*, 3rd edn. Mosby, London

Ford, M, Hennessey, I & Japp, A (2005) *Introduction to Clinical Examination*. Elsevier, Oxford

Gwinnutt, C (2006) *Clinical Anaesthesia*, 2nd edn. Blackwell Publishing, Oxford

Jevon, P (2001) *Advanced Cardiac Life Support*. Butterworth Heinemann, Oxford

Jevon, P (2007) Treating the Critically Ill Patient. Blackwell Publishing, Oxford.

Jevon, P & Cunnington, A (2006) Chest examination Part 3. Chest auscultation. *Nursing Times* **102**(46), 26–7

National Confidential Enquiry into Patient Outcome and Death (NCEPOD) (2005) *An Acute Problem*? NCEPOD, London.

Resuscitation Council UK (2000) *Cardiopulmonary Resuscitation: Guidelines for Clinical Practice and Training.* Resuscitation Council UK, London

Resuscitation Council UK (2004) *Recommended Minimum Equipment for In-Hospital Adult Resuscitation.* Resuscitation Council UK, London

Resuscitation Council UK (2006) *Advanced Life Support*, 5th edn. Resuscitation Council UK, London

Smith, G (2003) *ALERT Acute Life-Threatening Events Recognition and Treatment*, 2nd edn. University of Portsmouth, Portsmouth

Talley, N & O'Connor, S (2001) *Clinical Examination*, 4th edn. Blackwell Publishing, Oxford

# Respiratory Emergencies  2

## Kate Deacon

## INTRODUCTION

Respiratory emergencies can result from an array of different causes, from acute exacerbation of a long-term chronic respiratory disease to acute traumatic injury. In the UK one in five deaths are caused by respiratory disease. In 2004 more people died from respiratory disease (117,000) than from ischaemic heart disease (106,000) (British Thoracic Society, 2006). Once changes in the coding for deaths caused by pneumonia are taken into account, mortality rates from respiratory disease seen in 2004 have changed little in 20 years (British Thoracic Society, 2006).

Large socio-economic effects are seen in mortality rates for respiratory diseases, more than for any other type of disease. Social class inequality is estimated to be associated with 40% of respiratory deaths (British Thoracic Society, 2006).

The burden for the NHS of respiratory disease is a significant one. In English NHS hospitals in 2004/2005 there were 845,000 inpatient admissions for respiratory disease (7% of admissions); 550,000 of these were emergency admissions (13% of emergency admissions) (British Thoracic Society, 2006). In 2004 the cost to the NHS of respiratory disease was calculated to be £3 billion with a total cost to the UK economy of £6.6 billion (British Thoracic Society, 2006).

## LEARNING OUTCOMES

At the end of the chapter the reader will be able to:

❏ define respiratory failure,
❏ outline pulse oximetry and arterial blood gas (ABG) analysis,
❏ discuss the treatment of chronic obstructive pulmonary disease (COPD),
❏ discuss the treatment of asthma,
❏ discuss the treatment of pneumonia,
❏ discuss the treatment of acute respiratory distress syndrome (ARDS),
❏ discuss the treatment of pneumothorax.

## RESPIRATORY FAILURE

'Respiratory failure is defined as a failure to maintain adequate gas exchange and is characterised by abnormalities in arterial blood gas tensions' (British Thoracic Society Standards of Care Committee, 2002). Respiratory failure is split into two types, relating to the abnormalities seen in the arterial blood gases (ABGs). These are described in Table 2.1.

In type 1 (hypoxic) respiratory failure, ventilation is adequate but there is a problem with the exchange of oxygen. It is caused by a mismatch between ventilation and perfusion (V/Q mismatch). That is, the areas of the lung that are well ventilated are not well perfused with blood or vice versa.

Type 2 respiratory failure is caused by inadequate ventilation. As insufficient air reaches the areas of gas exchange, both $PaO_2$ and $PaCO_2$ are deranged.

Having an awareness of the effect of the type of respiratory failure a patient is experiencing is essential in ensuring that an appropriate method of monitoring oxygenation is employed.

**Table 2.1** Types 1 and 2 respiratory failure

| Type 1 respiratory failure | Type 2 respiratory failure |
| --- | --- |
| $PaO_2$ <8.0 kPa | $PaO_2$ <8.0 kPa |
| $PaCO_2$ normal or low | $PaCO_2$ >6.0 kPa |

Source: British Thoracic Society (2008).

## PULSE OXIMETRY AND ARTERIAL BLOOD GAS ANALYSIS

Pulse oximetry (Figure 2.1) is a non-invasive method for assessing the oxygen saturation of haemoglobin in the peripheral circulation ($SpO_2$ which has a direct correlation to arterial oxygen saturation ($SaO_2$)). It involves a probe that usually sits on the end of a finger; a combination of red and infrared light is used to calculate how well haemoglobin is saturated with oxygen (Jevon & Ewens, 2007). It is one of the physiological observations that the National Institute for Health and Clinical Excellence (NICE) Short Clinical Guidelines Technical Team (2007) have recently recommended should be taken as standard (see Chapter 11 in this volume).

Pulse oximetry is non-invasive, cheap and fairly simple to use; however, one should be aware that it does not provide information about the level of $CO_2$ in the patients blood, which would render it less suitable for use in patients with type 2 respiratory failure. For these measurements an ABG sample will need to be taken. Either samples can be obtained from a one-off arterial 'stab' using syringe and needle or an arterial line can be sighted

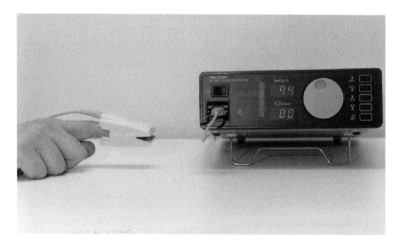

**Figure 2.1** A pulse oximetry monitor with finger probe

---

**Box 2.1 Normal arterial blood gas values**

| | |
|---|---|
| pH | 7.35–7.45 |
| $PaCO_2$ | 35–45 mmHg (as well as kPa) |
| $PaO_2$ | 10.0–14 kPa (75–105 mmHg) |
| Base excess | −2 mmol/+2 mmol |
| $HCO_3$ | 22–26 mmol/l |
| $SaO_2$ | 95–100% |

---

which has a port to allow blood samples to be taken. Taking arterial stab samples requires a level of skill and can be very uncomfortable for the patient; consideration should therefore be given to sighting an arterial line if frequent samples are required. Box 2.1 shows normal ABG values. Note that these values are for a healthy adult; those with chronic respiratory disease may have varied baseline values. Analysis of ABG results is described in detail elsewhere (Jevon & Ewens, 2007).

## CHRONIC OBSTRUCTIVE PULMONARY DISEASE (COPD)

COPD is an internationally recognised term that describes a spectrum of disease processes characterised by a chronic and progressive reduction in airflow. Although there may be an element of reversibility, most of the respiratory impairment is permanent and affects the upper airways, lung parenchyma and pulmonary circulation (Francis, 2006).

Specific diseases such as chronic bronchitis and emphysema are common causes of COPD; however, a small number have a diagnosis of emphysema without it progressing to a diagnosis of COPD (Selby, 2002). Also, whereas many smokers show symptoms of chronic bronchitis not all will develop the permanent airflow restriction of COPD as many will find that their symptoms disappear when they give up smoking (British Thoracic Society, 1997; Francis, 2006). Guidelines on the management of COPD have been published by NICE (NICE, 2004) and the Department of Health states that a National Service Framework for COPD will be published in 2008.

**Incidence**

At least 600,000 people in the UK have a diagnosis of COPD, a prevalence of 1%. However, one must be cognisant that diagnosis is usually made relatively late when definite symptoms have appeared (Calverly & Bellamy, 2000). In particular, smokers often ignore a persistent cough as simply being a side effect of the habit (Fehrenbach, 2002). In England alone in 2004 over 1 million hospital bed days were accounted for by COPD, and in the same year in the UK 27,478 people died from COPD, 23% of all respiratory deaths (British Thoracic Society, 2006). There is a strong socio-economic risk for COPD, with men of 20–64 years in manual unskilled occupations being 14 times more likely to die from COPD than those in professional ones (British Thoracic Society, 2006).

**Pathogenesis**

Chronic bronchitis is a state of mucus hypersecretion, defined as a productive cough on most days for 3 months for 2 consecutive years (without alternative explanation) (Bourke, 2003). The airways of chronic bronchitic patients have mucus-gland hypertrophy and excess goblet cells. The accumulation of mucus and the presence of infection can aggravate airway obstruction.

Emphysema causes airflow obstruction from damage to the alveoli, the walls of which are broken down and become distended. This may follow a pattern known as centrilobular, where the distended air spaces are those immediately next to the terminal bronchiole with more distal ones intact, or panacinar, where distension is spread throughout the acinus from the terminal bronchiole to the distal spaces (see Figure 2.2) (Bourke, 2003; Halpin, 2003).

Panacinar emphysema is the characteristic pattern seen in patients with alpha-1 ($\alpha$-1) anti-trypsin deficiency (Bourke, 2003). The terminal airways have no cartilage to keep them open and depend on the support of surrounding alveoli for this. Support is lost with the destruction of alveolar walls and the airways collapse during expiration, which leads to air trapping. With the

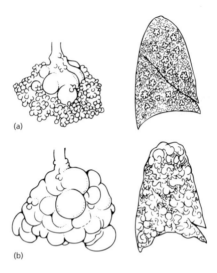

**Figure 2.2** Views of a lobule (left) and whole lung section (right) in (a) centrilobular and (b) panacinar emphysema

destruction of alveolar walls capillary blood supply is also lost, leading to ventilation/perfusion mismatch.

**Causes**

The single most important cause of COPD is cigarette smoking (British Thoracic Society, 1997; Bourke, 2003; Halpin, 2003). According to the British Thoracic Society COPD Consortium (2007) smoking is responsible for 95% of cases. COPD can develop in non-smokers but this is rare. Although nearly all COPD patients have smoked, only about 15% of smokers go on to develop clinically significant COPD (British Thoracic Society, 1997).

An inherited deficiency of the anti-protease α-1 anti-trypsin is associated with the development of severe emphysema with the risk being much increased in those with the deficiency who smoke (Global Initiative for Chronic Obstructive Lung Disease, 2006). A deficiency of α-1 anti-trypsin causes an imbalance

---

**Box 2.2 Risk factors for COPD**

Genes
Exposure to particles
  Tobacco smoke
  Occupational dusts, organic and inorganic
  Indoor air pollution from heating and cooking with biomass
  in poorly ventilated dwellings
  Outdoor air pollution
Lung growth and development
Oxidative stress
Gender
Age
Respiratory infections
Socio-economic status
Nutrition
Comorbidities

Source: Global Initiative for Chronic Obstructive Lung
Disease (2006).

---

between proteases and anti-proteases that leads to proteolytic destruction of lung tissue. However, this deficiency is stated to account for only 1–2% of severe COPD (Bourke, 2003; Halpin, 2003). There may be other heritable factors that have not yet been identified. A number of other factors have been shown to be implicated in the development of COPD. These are summarised in Box 2.2.

### Clinical features

There is great variability in the symptoms experienced by patients for different severities of airflow obstruction and in the rate of disease progression. Many patients with mild airflow obstruction will be asymptomatic (Halpin, 2003). Initially symptoms may be mild and intermittent but become more severe and continuous with severe airflow obstruction. The key symptoms of COPD are cough, wheeze and breathlessness (Halpin, 2003).

Chronic cough and sputum production are caused by mucus hypersecretion and infective exacerbations are commonly seen, which cause purulent secretions (Bourke, 2003). The patient often does not notice shortness of breath until a significant amount of respiratory function has been permanently lost, especially in those with a sedentary lifestyle; deterioration is usually gradual over a number of years (Bourke, 2003).

### Investigations

NICE (2004), in their clinical guidance on the management of COPD, recommended the following investigations for all suspected COPD patients:

- spirometry,
- chest X-ray,
- calculation of body mass index (BMI).

Further investigations may be necessary in some instances, as outlined in Table 2.2.

### Diagnosis

There is not one specific test for COPD and diagnosis is made from the overall clinical picture. NICE (2004) state that a diagnosis of COPD should be considered in patients who:

- are over 35;
- are smokers or ex-smokers;
- have any of these symptoms:
  - exertional breathlessness,
  - chronic cough,
  - regular sputum production,
  - frequent winter bronchitis;
- have no clinical symptoms of asthma.

Clinical features that may differentiate between asthma and COPD can be seen in Table 2.3.

**Table 2.2** Further investigations for COPD

| Investigation | Role |
|---|---|
| Serial domiciliary peak-flow measurements | To exclude asthma if diagnostic doubt remains |
| $\alpha$-1 Anti-trypsin | If early-onset, minimal smoking history or family history |
| Transfer factor for carbon monoxide (TLCO) | To investigate symptoms that seem disproportionate to the spirometric impairment |
| CT scan of the thorax | To investigate symptoms that seem disproportionate to the spirometric impairment |
| | To investigate abnormalities seen on a chest radiograph |
| | To assess suitability for surgery |
| ECG | To assess cardiac status if there are features of cor pulmonale |
| Echocardiogram | To assess cardiac status if there are features of cor pulmonale |
| Pulse oximetry | To assess need for oxygen therapy |
| | If cyanosis or cor pulmonale is present, or if $FEV_1$ <50% predicted |
| Sputum culture | To identify organisms if sputum is persistently present and purulent |

Source: NICE (2004).
$FEV_1$, forced expiratory volume in 1 s.

**Table 2.3** Clinical features of COPD and asthma

| | COPD | Asthma |
|---|---|---|
| Smoker or ex-smoker | Nearly all | Possibly |
| Symptoms under age 35 | Rare | Common |
| Chronic productive cough | Common | Uncommon |
| Breathlessness | Persistent and progressive | Variable |
| Night-time waking with breathlessness and/or wheeze | Uncommon | Common |
| Significant diurnal or day-to-day variability of symptoms | Uncommon | Common |

Source: NICE (2004).

If COPD seems likely from the above then spirometry should be performed to confirm airway obstruction. Airway obstruction is defined as (NICE, 2004; Global Initiative for Chronic Obstructive Lung Disease, 2006):

- forced expiratory volume in 1 s ($FEV_1$) <80% predicted,
- and $FEV_1$/forced vital capacity <0.7.

**Treatment**

In the UK guidance for COPD treatment is provided by the NICE clinical guidelines of 2004. Within this extensive guidance, recommendations are given for management of the chronic symptoms of mild, moderate and severe COPD as well as recommendations for acute exacerbations treated in hospital or at home.

- Assess the patient following the ABCDE approach (Chapter 1). Evaluate MEWS score and alert medics/outreach if necessary (see p. 298).
- Sit the patient in an upright position and administer oxygen. All critically ill patients should receive oxygen, including COPD patients. Caution should be exercised in COPD patients who have previously retained $CO_2$ in whom high concentration of oxygen may precipitate respiratory failure; the aim is to maintain oxygen saturations at 90–92%. (Resuscitation Council UK, 2006). Commence pulse oximetry.
- Administer nebulised bronchodilators; intravenous theophyllines may also be required.
- Assess the need for non-invasive ventilation, such as BiPAP (Bi level positive airways pressure).
- Monitor the patient's level of consciousness using AVPU and undertake regular pupillary assessment; if the patient's conscious level starts to deteriorate, for example drowsiness, they may becoming hypoxic or hypercapnoeic.
- If respiratory status is compromised, summon expert help immediately as tracheal intubation and mechanical ventilation may be required; whilst awaiting for help, provide ventilation as required.

- Insert a wide-bore intravenous cannula (e.g. 14 gauge) and obtain blood sample for relevant investigations, including full blood count, urea and electrolytes, liver-function tests and glucose.
- Ensure the following investigations are performed:
  - chest X-ray,
  - ABG (with record of inspired oxygen content),
  - ECG,
  - full blood count, urea and electrolytes,
  - Theophylline level if patient taking drug prior to admission,
  - sputum sample for microscopy and culture if purulent.

(NICE, 2004)

## ASTHMA

'Asthma is a condition which is characterised by episodes of reversible airway narrowing, associated with contraction of smooth muscle within the airway wall' (Weinberger, 2004). Various definitions such as this exist which describe the key characteristics of the disease; however, there isn't one agreed definition (BTS & SIGN, 2008).

There is considerable variation between patients in the severity of episodes experienced and the overall course of the disease. For some patients their illness is well controlled and they are asymptomatic between acute attacks whereas for others the illness can progress to a state of irreversible airway obstruction (Bourke, 2003).

### Incidence

There are 5.2 million people in the UK with asthma; of these 1.1 million are children and 4.1 million are adults (Asthma UK, 2004). Although the number of children with asthma has fallen since a peak in the 1990s the number of adults with asthma has risen, with an increase of 400,000 between 2001 and 2004. Asthma caused 69,000 hospital admissions and 1400 deaths in the UK in 2002 (Asthma UK, 2004).

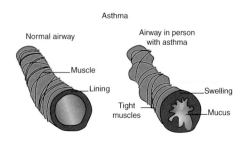

**Figure 2.3** A healthy bronchus and an asthmatic bronchus

### Pathogenesis

Asthma is characterised by episodes of reversible airway obstruction where hypersensitivity to certain triggers sets off an inflammatory response during which mucus is released and the muscles of the bronchi constrict (see Figure 2.3). The inflammatory process involves infiltration of the airway walls by various immune cells, oedema, hypertrophy of mucus glands and damage to the airway epithelial wall. This airway remodelling from persistent inflammation can lead to permanent fibrotic damage (Selby, 2002).

### Clinical features

During an exacerbation patients will often have wheeze (the cardinal sign of asthma) and reduced lung function, measured by peak flow or spirometry. The symptoms experienced by asthma patients are not exclusive to asthma and note should be taken of the manner in which these symptoms tend to be experienced (see Box 2.4).

### Investigations and diagnosis

Apart from the signs and symptoms described above certain other information would lead towards a suspicion of asthma (BTS & SIGN, 2008):

- personal or family history of asthma or other atopic condition,
- worsening of symptoms after exposure to recognised triggers (pollen, dust, etc.),

---

**Box 2.4 Asthma symptoms**

**Symptoms experienced**
Wheeze
Shortness of breath
Chest tightness
Cough
**Nature of symptoms**
Variable
Intermittent
Worse at night
Provoked by triggers including exercise and early morning

Source: British Thoracic Society and Scottish Intercollegiate
Guidelines Network (2008).

---

- Worsening of symptoms after taking aspirin, non-steroidal anti-inflammatory drugs or beta-blockers.

Airway obstruction can be measured objectively by assessing peak expiratory flow (PEF) and forced expiratory volume in 1 s ($FEV_1$). However, readings may be normal between acute attacks and a one-off measurement will not be able to demonstrate the variability (spontaneous or in response to treatment) that is characteristic of asthma. One or both of PEF or $FEV_1$ should be assessed and variability calculated, looking for a change of 60 litres/min for PEF, and a change of 400 mls for $FEV_1$ is seen as highly suggestive of asthma (BTS & SIGN, 2008).

**Treatment**

The guideline on the management of asthma provided by the British Thoracic Society (BTS) and the Scottish Intercollegiate Guidelines Network (SIGN) is a comprehensive evidence-based guide that was updated in May 2008 and is supported by a number of organisations including Asthma UK. Guidance is provided relating to initial diagnosis, long term management, and management of acute exacerbations and follow up care. A number of algorithms are provided for the management of acute asthma in infants, children and adults, in different settings and for varying levels of severity. The full guideline can be accessed through the British Thoracic society's web site at www.brit-thoracic.org.uk.

If the patient presents with acute shortness of breath the following treatment is required:

- Assess the patient following the ABCDE approach described in Chapter 1. Evaluate MEWS score and alert medics/outreach if necessary (see p. 298).
- Ensure the patient has a clear airway.
- Sit the patient in an upright position and administer oxygen.
- All critically ill patients should receive oxygen (exercise caution in COPD; see above)
- Commence pulse oximetry and perform ABG analysis.

Treatment interventions for an acute asthma attack are guided according to the severity of the attack. Box 2.5 defines the categories of severity.

The full BTS & SIGN (2008) guidance for the management of asthma addresses management in children and adults; in community and hospital settings. The guidance for management and monitoring of adults with severe asthma in hospital is summarised in box 2.6 below. Before a patient who has been admitted with severe acute asthma is discharged from hospital, it is essential that consideration be given not only to suitability for discharge but also patient follow up once in the community. (For recommendations regarding discharge and follow up see full guidance). Investigations of asthma deaths within the UK have highlighted inadequate management, monitoring and follow up as contributing factors for some patients (BTS & SIGN 2008). A previous admission for asthma, particularly in the last year is, one of a number of factors that were found to make a patient more likely to be at risk of suffering a fatal or near-fatal asthma attack (BTS & SIGN 2008).

## PNEUMONIA

Pneumonia is a term used to describe inflammation of the gas-exchange area of the lungs, usually as a result of infection (Bourke, 2003). Pneumonia may be community-acquired, developing

---

**Box 2.5 Categories of severity for acute asthma attacks (Taken from Annexe 4 of the 2008 BTS/SIGN Asthma Guidelines)**

**Features of severe acute asthma**

- Peak expiratory flow (PEF) 35–50% of best (use % of predicted if best unknown)
- Can't complete sentences in one breath
- Respirations $\Rightarrow$ 25 breaths/min.
- Pulse $\Rightarrow$ 110 beats/min.

**Features of life threatening asthma**

- PEF <33% of best or predicted
- $SpO_2$ <92%
- Silent chest, cyanosis or feeble respiratory effort
- Bradycardia, dysrhythmia or hypotension
- Exhaustion, confusion or coma.
  - *If a patient has any life-threatening feature, measure arterial blood gas. No other investigations are needed for immediate management*
  - *Blood gas markers of a life threatening attack:*
  - *Normal PaCO2-(4.6–6 kPa)*
  - *Severe hypoxia- $Pao_2$ < 8.0 kpa irrespective of treatment with oxygen*
  - *A low pH (or high $H^+$)*

*(Caution patients with severe or life threatening attacks may not be distressed and may not have all these abnormalities. The presences of any should alert the doctor).*

**Features of near fatal asthma**

- Raised PaCO2
- Requiring IPPV with raised inflation pressures

---

in those who are previously fit and healthy or those with a preexisting chronic condition such as COPD, or it may be hospital-acquired, where a patient develops pneumonia 2 or more days after being admitted to hospital for another reason (Francis, 2006). Factors relating to the patient, the environment and the organism interact in the development of pneumonia (Bourke, 2003).

**Box 2.6 Management of severe asthma in adults in hospital (Taken from Annexe 4 of the 2008 BTS/SIGN Asthma Guidelines)**

**Immediate treatment**

- Oxygen 40–60% ($CO_2$ retention is not usually aggravated by oxygen therapy in asthma)
- Salbutamol 5 mg or Terbutaline 10 mg via an oxygen driven nebuliser
- Ipraprotium bromide 0.5 mg via an oxygen driven nebuliser
- Prednisolone tablets 40–50 mgs or IV hydrocortisone 100 mg or both if very ill
- No sedatives of any kind
- Chest X-ray only if Pneumothorax or consolidation are suspected or patient requires IPPV
  - **If life threatening features are present**:
  - Discuss with senior clinician and ICU team
  - Add IV magnesium sulphate 1.2–2 g infusion over 20 minutes (unless already given)
  - Give nebulised $\beta_2$ agonist more frequently e.g. Salbutamol 5 mg up to every 15–30 minutes or 10 mg continuously hourly.

**Subsequent management**

IF PATIENT IS IMPROVING, continue:

- 40–60% oxygen
- Prednisolone 40–50 mgs daily or IV Hydrocortisone 100 mg 6 hourly
- Nebulised $\beta_2$ agonist and Ipraprotium 4–6 hourly

IF PATIENT NOT IMPROVING AFTER 15–30 MINS:

- Continue oxygen and steroids
- Give nebulised $\beta_2$ agonist more frequently e.g. Salbutamol 5 mg up to every 15–30 minutes or 10 mg continuously hourly.
- Continue Ipraprotium 0.5 mg 4–6 hourly until patient is improving

IF PATIENT IS STILL NOT IMPROVING:

- Discuss with senior clinician and ICU team
- IV magnesium sulphate 1.2–2 g over 20 mins (unless already given)

- Senior clinician may consider the use of IV $\beta_2$ agonist or IV aminophylline or consider progression to IPPV

**Monitoring**

- Repeat measurement of PEF 15–30 minutes after starting treatment
- Oximetry: maintain SpO2 >92%
- Repeat blood gas measurements within 2 ours of starting treatment if:
  ○ Initial PaO2 <8.0 kpa unless subsequent SpO2 >92%
  ○ PaCO2 normal or raised
  ○ Patient deteriorates
- Chart PEF before and after giving and at least 4 times daily throughout hospital stay

  *Transfer to ICU accompanied by a doctor prepared to intubate if*:

  - Deteriorating PEF, worsening or persisting hypoxia or hypercapnia
  - Exhaustion, feeble respiration, confusion or drowsiness
  - Coma or respiratory arrest

**Incidence**

In the UK 34,000 people died of pneumonia in 2004, accounting for 29% of respiratory deaths (British Thoracic Society, 2006). In women pneumonia is the largest respiratory cause of death, accounting for 35% of respiratory deaths.

**Causes and pathogenesis**

Pneumonia can be caused by bacterial, viral and less frequently fungal organisms; it can also be caused by aspiration of gastric contents. The pathogenesis depends on the causative factor.

- Aspiration of gastric contents causes inflammation of the lung affected and can significantly inactivate surfactant, leading to alveolar collapse. Acid from gastric secretions can damage the airways and particles can cause an airway obstruction.
- Bacterial pneumonia produces an inflammatory process at the alveolar membrane; this causes oedema and stasis of blood,

which leads to atelectasis because the alveoli fill with exudate, and blood.

- Viral pneumonia causes interstitial inflammation that initially affects the bronchial epithelium but then spreads to the alveoli.
- Fungal pneumonias are less common and tend to affect people who are immunocompromised

(Source: Dunn, 2005)

## Clinical features

Patients with pneumonia will usually present the following clinical features:

- cough,
- purulent sputum,
- fever,
- pleuritic pain,
- dyspnoea.

On chest examination crackles, dullness or bronchial breathing are also suggestive of pneumonia; elderly patients may present with confusion (Bourke, 2003).

## Investigations

- Chest X-ray: to aid diagnosis, exclude any underlying disease and assess response to treatment.
- Blood cultures: to indicate septicaemia/bacteraemia.
- Haematology and biochemistry: useful in assessing the severity of disease.
- Sputum sample: for culture, sensitivity, Gram stain and Ziehl–Nielsen stain for tuberculosis.
- Urine antigen tests: for *Streptococcus pneumoniae* and *Legionella* (British Thoracic Society Pneumonia Guidelines Committee, 2004).
- White cell count: this will be raised in bacterial pneumonia.

(Sources: Bourke, 2003; Dunn, 2005)

## Diagnosis

Diagnosis is made on the basis of clinical presentation. A productive cough may or may not be present; sputum that is yellow, green, rusty or blood-stained is likely to indicate a bacterial cause (Dunn, 2005). *Streptococcus pneumoniae* (often known as pneumococcus) is the most common form of pneumonia (Dunn, 2005).

### Treatment

Guidance from the British Thoracic Society Pneumonia Guidelines Committee (2004) recommends the use of the CRB-65 score (see Box 2.7) to determine where to manage patients with community-acquired pneumonia when in hospital.

If the patient presents with acute shortness of breath the following treatment is required.

- Assess the patient following the ABCDE approach (Chapter 1). Evaluate MEWS score and alert medics/outreach if necessary (see p. 298).
- Sit the patient in an upright position and administer oxygen. Exercise caution in COPD with previous episode of $CO_2$ retention. Commence pulse oximetry and perform ABG analysis.
- Assess the need for non-invasive ventilation, such as BiPAP.

---

**Box 2.7 CURB-65 score and action for patients with community-acquired pneumonia**

**Any of . . .**
Confusion
Respiratory rate >30 breaths/min
Blood pressure (SBP <90 mmHg or DBP <60 mmHg)
Age ≥65 years
**Score 1 point for each feature present**
CRB-65 score 0: likely to be suitable for home treatment
CRB-65 score 1 or 2: consider hospital
CRB-65 score 3 or 4: urgent hospital admission

Source: British Thoracic Society (2004).
DBP, diastolic blood pressure; SBP, systolic blood pressure.
Note that the full name for this score is CURB-65, with the U standing for urea, which isn't always used, hence the use of CRB-65 in the text itself.

The British Thoracic Society Pneumonia Guidelines Committee (2004) guidance for the management of community-acquired pneumonia for patients needing treatment in hospital recommends the following.

- Patients should receive oxygen therapy with monitoring of $SaO_2$ and fraction of inspired oxygen ($FiO_2$), aiming for a $PaO_2$ of $\geq 8.0$ kPa and $SaO_2$ of $\geq 92\%$.
- Oxygen therapy in patients with pre-existing COPD complicated by ventilatory failure should be guided by repeated ABGs.
- Patients should be assessed for volume depletion and may require intravenous fluids.
- Temperature, pulse, respiratory rate, blood pressure, mental status, $SaO_2$ and inspired oxygen concentration should be monitored at least twice daily, more frequently in those with severe pneumonia or requiring regular oxygen therapy.
- C-reactive protein levels should be re-measured and chest X-ray repeated on patients who are not progressing satisfactorily.
- Most patients with non-severe pneumonia can be treated with oral antibiotics.
- Patients with severe pneumonia should be treated immediately after diagnosis with parenteral antibiotics.

The guidelines also offer further detailed advice about patients with community-acquired pneumonia managed in the community, follow-up planning and specific antibiotic advice (British Thoracic Society Pneumonia Guidelines Committee, 2004).

## ACUTE RESPIRATORY DISTRESS SYNDROME (ARDS)

ARDS is a severe form of acute respiratory failure that causes profound hypoxaemia. It is a syndrome rather than a specific disease brought about by a number of different illnesses or injuries. ARDS was first described in 1967 with the 'A' initially standing for adult as it was thought that it only occurred in adults. This has since been realised to be incorrect and the 'A' became acute in recognition of this (Morton et al., 2005). The recognition of ARDS gave an explanation for the deaths of some soldiers in the first and second world wars, and subsequent conflicts, who would become injured and survive their initial wounds and then die days later from respiratory failure (Bourke, 2003).

## Incidence

A UK study reported an incidence of ARDS of 4.3 in 100,000 population per year, which is in line with a previous UK study. The authors report that these figures are also similar to recent studies in other countries (Dixon & Gunning, 2000).

## Pathogenesis

In ARDS there is inflammation and injury to the alveolar/capillary membrane, which increases capillary permeability and leads to permeability pulmonary oedema. The alveoli become filled with a protein-rich exudate containing various inflammatory cells. The pathological process moves through exudative, inflammatory and fibroproliferative or reparative stages. This causes impaired gas exchange, atelectasis, V/Q mismatch, shunting and the severely reduced compliance that is synonymous with ARDS, which leads to refractory hypoxaemia (Bourke, 2003; Taylor, 2005; Leaver & Evans, 2007).

## Causes

An extensive list (over 60) of causes of ARDS has been identified, because any illness or injury that can cause a systemic inflammatory response can potentially cause ARDS (Taylor, 2005). However, risk for developing ARDS has been shown to be particularly high for sepsis, septic shock, trauma and aspiration of gastric contents. The highest risk is seen in septic shock of a pulmonary source, which carries an ARDS incidence rate of 48% (Leaver & Evans, 2007).

## Clinical features

The clinical features of ARDS usually start to develop within 12–48 h of the precipitating event. The patient presents in a state of respiratory distress with worsening dyspnoea and tachypnoea. Initial ABGs reveal a respiratory alkalosis secondary to tachypnoea: very low $PO_2$, raised pH and normal or low $PCO_2$. The hypoxaemia worsens and shows a poor response to oxygen therapy, as the patient tires their $PCO_2$ starts to rise and their ABG picture becomes one of respiratory acidosis. On chest X-ray diffuse bilateral infiltrates can be seen (in the absence of cardiogenic pulmonary oedema) (Bourke, 2003; Taylor, 2005).

### Investigations

Investigations aim to define the extent of lung injury, aid diagnosis of ARDS and elucidate precipitating factors. The list below summarises the recommended investigations with their rationale (from Leaver & Evans, 2007).

- Chest X-ray: to assess for diffuse bilateral infiltrates.
- ABG: to establish the severity of hypoxaemia.
- Echocardiography: to differentiate lung injury from cardiogenic pulmonary oedema.
- CT thorax: to aid identification of pulmonary precipitating factors, for example lung abscess.
- Fibreoptic bronchoscopy and bronchiolar lavage: to help exclude infection in patients not responding to treatment.

### Diagnosis

In 1994 the American-European Consensus Conference (AECC) proposed diagnostic criteria for acute lung injury (ALI) and ARDS. Although the criteria are not without criticism they are still commonly used (Morton et al., 2005; Taylor, 2005). The AECC criteria are shown in Table 2.4.

### Treatment

Treatment in ARDS needs to focus on treating the precipitating factor as well as supporting the respiratory system. The aim is to try and maintain oxygenation and perfusion via ventilation and fluid management. Management should also aim to minimise sources of sepsis by removal of known sources (e.g. ischaemic bowel, abscess) and trying to prevent new infection (Bourke, 2003; Taylor, 2005).

The cornerstone of management for ARDS is mechanical ventilation (discussed below). A number of other interventions have been proposed; a variety of different types of drugs have been

**Table 2.4** American-European Consensus Conference (AECC) criteria for acute lung injury (ALI) and ARDS

|  | **ALI** | **ARDS** |
| --- | --- | --- |
| Timing | Acute onset | Acute onset |
| Chest X-ray | Bilateral infiltrates on frontal chest radiograph | Bilateral infiltrates on frontal chest radiograph |
| PCWP | <18 mmHg and/or no clinical evidence of left-atrial hypertension (CHF) | <18 mmHg and/or no clinical evidence of left-atrial hypertension (CHF) |
| $PaO_2/FiO_2$ ratio (regardless of PEEP level) | ≤300 mmHg | ≤200 mmHg |

CHF, congestive heart failure; PCWP, pulmonary capillary wedge pressure; PEEP, positive end-expiratory pressure.

tested in the treatment of ARDS. However, a Cochrane review (Adhikari et al., 2004) concluded that although some small studies had shown some degree of benefit the overall conclusion was that there was insufficient evidence of any survival benefit of pharmacotherapies in ARDS. Various interventions for mechanical ventilation have been proposed and are summarised below.

- Lung protection: the distribution of pathological changes in ARDS means that there is a risk of some areas of the lung being distended and exposed to high pressure that can result in volutrauma and barotraumas. Support has been found in terms of a significant reduction in mortality rates, for ventilating with a low tidal volume (6 ml/kg). Allowing the $PaCO_2$ to rise, in order to use small ventilation volumes to protect the lungs, is known as permissive hypercapnia, which has been seen as acceptable in practice as long as $PaO_2$ is acceptable and pH remains above 7.2 (Leaver & Evans, 2007).
- The use of positive end-expiratory pressure (PEEP) recruits small airways, prevents alveolar collapse and improves V/Q mismatch by reducing shunting. However, research that has compared a high and low setting of PEEP showed no significant effect on mortality or other outcome measures (Leaver & Evans, 2007).

- Nitric oxide is a vasodilator and when inhaled reduces pulmonary vascular resistance, bringing about a noticeable oxygenation improvement in most patients. However, the effect is transitory and its use does not significantly reduce mortality or duration of ventilation, therefore, it is not recommended for routine use (Leaver & Evans, 2007).
- Extra-corporeal membrane oxygenation (ECMO) involves attaching the patient to a circuit in which their blood passes through a filter that takes over the role of oxygenating the blood and removing carbon dioxide. It is an expensive treatment that is only available in regional centres. Evidence does not currently exist as to the effect on mortality rates of transferring a patient with ARDS to a centre providing ECMO as opposed to providing conventional ventilation in the unit they are in. However, a trial examining this has been carried out (the Cesar trial) and results are currently being analysed.

## PNEUMOTHORAX

The term pneumothorax describes the presence of air in the pleural space. Most commonly, air enters the space internally from a breach in the visceral pleura but can enter from the outside following traumatic chest injury (Selby, 2002). A pneumothorax may be classified as spontaneous or traumatic in origin. Spontaneous pneumothoraces can be primary, where they are not related to any pre-existing lung disease, or secondary, where they are (Bourke, 2003).

### Incidence

In the UK, hospital admission rates for combined primary and secondary spontaneous pneumothorax are reported as 5.8 in 100,000 per year for women and 16.7 in 100,000 per year for men. A bimodal age distribution pattern can be seen such that there is a peak in the younger age group (15–34 years) and a peak in the older age group (>55 years) that corresponds respectively with primary and secondary spontaneous pneumothorax (Gupta et al., 2000).

### Pathogenesis

Spontaneous primary pneumothoraces are usually caused by the rupture of a subpleural bleb or bullae. This is most commonly seen in tall young men who have been previously healthy. As intra-alveolar pressure is higher than intra-pleural pressure, air readily rushes into the pleural space once there has been a breach, in order to equalise pressure. This occurs more frequently in men than women by a ratio of 3:1. Smoking increases the risk of primary spontaneous pneumothorax by nine times in women and 22 times in men (Bourke, 2003). A number of conditions are associated with secondary spontaneous pneumothorax, particularly emphysema and asthma, but other conditions such as tuberculosis, sarcoidosis, cystic fibrosis and staphylococcal pneumonia may also be involved (Jenkins, 2005).

Sometimes the hole that has allowed air into the pleural space will occur in such a way that it acts as a flap or valve, so that it opens during inspiration, allowing air into the pleural space, but then the flaps shut during expiration so that none of the air can escape back out. With each breath more air accumulates in the pleural space, squashing the lung itself. This is known as a tension pneumothorax and is a life-threatening situation. If left untreated the pressure will continue to increase, causing mediastinal shift and a decrease in venous return and cardiac output. This could lead to pulseless electrical activity (PEA) cardiac arrest which would only be resolved by removing the trapped air and thereby relieving the pressure.

In traumatic pneumothorax, air may enter the pleural space internally caused by the puncture of a fractured rib or externally from a penetrating chest injury. Iatrogenic (doctor-induced) pneumothorax may occur as a complication of a medical procedure such as insertion of a central venous catheter via the subclavian vein (Bourke, 2003).

### Clinical features

The main clinical features of pneumothorax are breathlessness and pleuritic pain. The degree of breathlessness is determined by the underlying respiratory health and the size of the pneumothorax. A fit and healthy young adult may be able to cope with a pneumothorax that in an older patient with underlying lung disease could cause severe respiratory distress (Selby, 2002; Bourke, 2003).

On examination, reduced breath sounds, reduced chest expansion and hyper-resonance are signs of pneumothorax. Key clinical signs of tension pneumothorax are mediastinal shift and haemodynamic compromise (Selby, 2002).

### Investigation and diagnosis

Chest X-ray is the investigation to be carried out following clinical examination for the features described above. On X-ray a pneumothorax will show up as a black featureless area with no lung markings from the edge of the collapsed area to the chest wall (Bourke, 2003). Due to the urgent and life-threatening nature of tension pneumothorax, where haemodynamic compromise is observed clinical signs of tension pneumothorax should be checked for:

- Hyper-resonant hemi-thorax.
- Absent air entry of affected side.
- Tracheal deviation away from affected side.

### Treatment

If the patient presents with acute shortness of breath the following treatment is required.

- Assess the patient following the ABCDE approach (Chapter 1). Evaluate MEWS score and alert medics/outreach if necessary (see p. 298).
- Sit the patient in an upright position and administer a high concentration of oxygen (see above). Commence pulse oximetry and perform ABG analysis.
- Insert a wide-bore intravenous cannula (e.g. 14 gauge) and obtain a blood sample for routine investigations, for example full blood count, urea and electrolytes, and glucose.
- Monitor the patient's level of consciousness using the AVPU scale (Box 6.1) and undertake regular pupillary assessment

The appropriate treatment depends on the size of the pneumothorax.

- A small pneumothorax (<20% of hemithorax) that is not symptomatic may not require any action, as it will resolve spontaneously at the rate of 1–2% per day (Allibone, 2003). Prior to discharge patients need to be advised to return immediately to hospital if their condition deteriorates. Follow-up should be arranged to include chest X-ray and clinical examination to confirm that the pneumothorax has resolved and check for any underlying related pathology. Patients should be advised not to fly until at least 6 weeks after the pneumothorax has resolved because of the risk that the reduced air pressure will cause any small pockets of air still present to re-expand (Bourke, 2003).

- Air can be removed from the pleural space by aspiration; this is a less distressing process for the patient than insertion of an intercostal drainage tube. The area should first be numbed with local anaesthetic. A French 16-gauge cannula is inserted into the second intercostal space at the midclavicular line. Once in the correct position the needle is removed and a syringe attached via a three-way tap; air can then be drawn off. The success of the procedure should be confirmed with chest X-ray. Insertion of an intercostal drainage tube will become necessary if: the aspiration was not successful, a tension pneumothorax is present or there is a need to drain blood as well as remove air, as may be the case following trauma. (Bourke, 2003).

- Insertion of an intercostal chest drain tube can be a traumatic and distressing experience for the patient. It is therefore essential that they be given adequate explanation and reassurance throughout the procedure. A small dose of sedative such as intravenous midazolam 1–2 mg may be needed for a very anxious patient (Bourke, 2003). An aseptic technique needs to be employed. Before commencing the procedure the correct insertion site should be confirmed by reviewing the chest X-ray. Where fluid and air need to be drained the patient may require two drains, one apical and one basal, as fluid will settle with gravity and air will rise (Allibone, 2003). The usual position for insertion will be the mid-axillary line at the fourth, fifth or sixth intercostal space. The area should be well anaesthetised with lignocaine including the skin, muscle and parietal pleura (10–20 ml of 1% lignocaine) (Bourke, 2003). The skin is cut and a track for the chest tube is then created using blunt dissection with forceps; this track should be wide enough to allow the tube to slide in without force (Bourke, 2003). The tube is secured with a strong suture and connected to an underwater drainage system. This allows air to escape but prevents air from returning back up the tube. Throughout the procedure the nurse should monitor the patient's overall clinical picture, particularly their breathing, $SpO_2$ levels, haemodynamic state and general demeanour. The nurse should offer constant reassurance and explanation to the patient.

- Following insertion of a chest drain, the activity of the chest drain and condition of the patient should be monitored closely according to local policy, of which there is variation (Allibone, 2003). A rise and fall of the fluid level in the drainage bottle with breathing indicates that the tube is patent; bubbling indicates that air is draining. Impedance to drainage can cause tension pneumothorax or surgical emphysema; it is therefore important to make sure the tube is not kinked (Allibone, 2003). For this reason the tube should only be clamped when changing the drainage bottle or if the tubing has become accidentally disconnected (Mallet & Dougherty, 2000). This situation must be dealt with immediately; the tubes should not be left clamped.

## CONCLUSION

Respiratory failure can be caused by a vast number of respiratory illnesses; this chapter has highlighted five relatively common ones. Regardless of the cause of the failure each patient should initially be assessed to establish the seriousness of the situation using the ABCDE approach. Various methods of assessment and monitoring can be used which will give information as to the patient's oxygen level and the volumes that they are breathing. For some measurements a one-off reading will be useful but for many assessments, especially where there is an established history of chronic disease, it is essential to have a baseline for comparison with subsequent monitoring of trend. If a patient appears to be, or indicates that they are in any way, distressed with their breathing this is sufficient information to dictate that further investigation of the situation is required.

## REFERENCES

Adhikari, NK, Burns, KE & Meade, MO (2004) Pharmacologic therapies for adults with acute lung injury and acute respiratory distress syndrome. *Cochrane Database Systematic Review* 4, CD004477

Allibone, L (2003) Nursing management of chest drains. *Nursing Standard* **17**(22), 45–54

Asthma UK (2004) *Where Do We Stand? – Asthma in the UK Today.* Asthma UK, London

Bourke, SJ (2003) *Respiratory Medicine*, 6th edn. Blackwell Publishing, Oxford

British Thoracic Society (1997) BTS guidelines for the management of chronic obstructive pulmonary disease. *Thorax* (suppl.) **5**, 1–28

British Thoracic Society (2006) *The Burden of Lung Disease*, 2nd edn. British Thoracic Society, London

British Thoracic Society COPD Consortium (2007) *COPD Background*. www.brit-thoracic.org.uk/copd-background.html (accessed 22 August 2007). British Thoracic Society, London

British Thoracic Society Pneumonia Guidelines Committee (2004) *Guidelines for the Management of Community Acquired Pneumonia in Adults.* British Thoracic Society, London

British Thoracic Society and Scottish Intercollegiate Guidelines Network (2008) *British Guideline on the Management of Asthma – A National Clinical Guideline.* British Thoracic Society, London

British Thoracic Society Standards of Care Committee (2002) Non-invasive ventilation in acute respiratory failure. *Thorax* **57**, 192–211

Calverly, P & Bellamy, D (2000) The challenge of providing better care for patients with chronic obstructive pulmonary disease: the poor relation of airways obstruction? *Thorax* **55**(1), 78–82

Dixon, JM & Gunning, KEJ (2000) The incidence of ARDS, interim results of the East Anglian ARDS Registry. *Critical Care* **4** (suppl.), 130

Dunn, L (2005) Pneumonia: classification, diagnosis and nursing management. *Nursing Standard* **19**(42), 50–4

Fehrenbach, C (2002) Chronic obstrutive pulmonary disease. *Nursing Standard* **17**(10), 45–51

Francis, C (2006) *Respiratory Care*. Blackwell Publishing, Oxford

Global Initiative for Chronic Obstructive Lung Disease (2006) *Global Strategy for the Diagnosis, Management and Prevention of Chronic Obstructive Pulmonary Disease*. GOLD Executive Summary. *American Journal of Respiratory and Critical Care Medicine* **176**, 532–55

Gupta, D, Hansell, A, Nichols, T, Duong, T, Ayres, JG & Strachan, D (2000) Epidemiology of pneumothorax in England. *Thorax* **55**, 666–71

Halpin, DMG (2003) *Your Questions Answered – COPD*. Churchill Livingstone, Edinburgh

Jenkins, PF (2005) *Making Sense of the Chest X-Ray: A Hands on Guide*. Hodder Education, London

Jevon, P & Ewens, B (2007) *Monitoring the Critically Ill Patient*, 2nd edn. Blackwell Publishing, Oxford

Leaver, SK & Evans, TW (2007) Acute respiratory distress syndrome. *British Medical Journal* **335**, 389–94

Mallet, J & Dougherty, L (eds) (2000) *The Royal Marsden Hospital Handbook of Clinical Procedures*, 5th edn. Blackwell Publishing, Oxford

Morton, PG, Fontaine, DK, Hudak, CM & Gallo, BM (2005) *Critical Care Nursing – A Holistic Approach*, 8th edn. Lippincott Williams and Wilkins, Philadelphia, PA

NICE (2004) *Chronic Obstructive Pulmonary Disease – Management of Chronic Obstructive Pulmonary Disease in Adults in Primary and Secondary Care*. Clinical guidance 12. NICE, London

NICE Short Clinical Guidelines Technical Team (2007) *Acutely Ill Patients in Hospital – Recognition of and Response to Acute Illness in Adults in Hospital*. NICE, London

Resuscitation Council UK (2006) *Advanced Life Support*, 5th edn. Resuscitation Council UK, London

Selby, CD (2002) *Respiratory Medicine: an Illustrated Colour Text*. Churchill Livingstone, Edinburgh

Taylor, MM (2005) ARDS diagnosis and management. *Dimensions of Critical Care Nursing* **24**(5), 197–207

Weinberger, SE (2004) *Principles of Pulmonary Medicine*, 4th edn. Saunders, Philadelphia, PA

# Cardiac Emergencies

**3**

## Melanie Humphreys

### INTRODUCTION

Cardiovascular diseases exert a huge burden on individuals and society: coronary heart disease (CHD) is the single most common cause of death in the UK and other developed countries (British Heart Foundation, 2004). Improved clinical care has been responsible for around two-fifths of the decline in mortality from CHD in England and Wales over the past decade (Unal et al., 2004).

Startlingly, however, studies still suggest that many critically ill patients have cardiac arrest because of inadequate initial assessment and subsequent non-recognition of patient deterioration (Resuscitation Council UK, 2006). Sudden cardiac emergencies are particularly distressing and frightening, not only for patients but also for carers. Activity, levels of anxiety, speed of onset and previous experience may influence patients' perception of its severity.

Virtually every pathological process affecting the heart can lead to a critical cardiac event, and commonly sudden death. Therefore a good understanding of emergency cardiac events and their immediate management is essential in reducing this risk. Through a structured approach of assessment, initiating investigations, treatment and delivering appropriate care, potential life-threatening cardiac events can be identified, alerting medical staff immediately to these situations, and ensuring that the most appropriate evidence-based treatment strategies are adopted.

The aim of this chapter is to allow the reader to understand the treatment of cardiac emergencies.

## LEARNING OUTCOMES

At the end of this chapter the reader will be able to:

❏ describe the causes, presentation and treatment of left-ventricular failure (LVF) and the immediate care of this group of patients,

❏ discuss the concept of acute coronary syndromes (ACSs),

❏ outline the priorities of caring for a patient having an acute myocardial infarction (MI),

❏ describe cardiac-arrest rhythms and their immediate treatment,

❏ discuss the aetiology of cardiac tamponade and cardiogenic shock,

❏ describe the priorities of nursing care for patients with acute cardiac emergencies.

## LEFT-VENTRICULAR FAILURE (LVF)

Heart failure is a major cause of morbidity and mortality in the Western world. In the UK, it is estimated to account for 5% of all hospital admissions: approximately 100,000 each year (National Institute for Health and Clinical Excellence, NICE, 2003). Heart failure affects 3–20 people per 1000, although this number exceeds 100 per 1000 in those aged 65 or over. It is estimated to occur in 900,000 people per year in the UK and the average age is 76 years (NICE, 2003). The incidence of heart failure is increasing because of the ageing population, and advancements in cardiac care particularly cardiac reperfusion.

Advancement in treatments of acute myocardial infarction (MI), such as thrombolysis and emergency coronary angioplasty, leads to survival in patients with impaired left-ventricular function. LVF is characterised by the inability of the left ventricle to deliver sufficient oxygenated blood to meet the needs of tissues, either at rest or during exercise. Congestive heart failure (CHF), also called congestive cardiac failure (CCF), is a condition that can result from any structural or functional cardiac disorder that impairs the ability of the heart to fill with, or pump, a sufficient amount of blood throughout the body. Heart failure is often undiagnosed due to a lack of a universally agreed definition and difficulties in diagnosis, particularly when the condition is considered 'mild'. Even with the best therapy, heart failure is associated with an annual mortality of 10% (Neubauer, 2007).

There are many different ways to categorise heart failure, including:

- the side of the heart involved (left heart failure or right heart failure),
- whether the abnormality is due to contraction or relaxation of the heart (systolic heart failure or diastolic heart failure),
- whether the abnormality is due to low cardiac output or low systemic vascular resistance (low-output heart failure or high-output heart failure)

Typology includes the following.

- *Acute, sudden onset*: new presentation; this may be the result of acute MI, arrhythmias, valvular disease or infection.
- *Chronic, gradual onset*: symptoms gradually progress and can be very debilitating.
- *Acute on chronic*: acute onset in patients with chronic disease.

Regardless of the category, severe acute heart failure is a medical emergency, and effective management requires an assessment of the underlying cause, improvement of the haemodynamic status, relief of pulmonary congestion and improved tissue oxygenation. Clinical and radiographic assessment of these patients provides a guide to severity and prognosis (Millane et al., 2000).

### Causes

The usual pathological processes affecting the heart can make heart failure deadly: arterial plaque, raised blood pressure, stress, smoking, old age, a lack of exercise, overworked heart and obesity. In a genetic family history of CHF, the cause is a weak heart with thinner muscle walls than usual, and often weakened further by one or more of the contributing factors (see below).

Arterial plaque lines the inside of the arteries that supply the heart and the rest of the body, meaning that less blood gets to the heart itself, as well as the heart having to work harder to push blood through the thinner systemic arteries. The result can be arrhythmias causing inefficient blood pumping and a tired heart.

Causes and contributing factors to LVF include the following:

- genetic family history of CHF,
- ischaemic heart disease/MI (coronary artery disease),
- thyrotoxicosis (hyperthyroidism),
- arrhythmia,
- hypertension,
- cardiac fibrosis,
- coarctation of the aorta,
- aortic stenosis/regurgitation,
- mitral regurgitation,
- pulmonary stenosis/pulmonary hypertension/pulmonary embolism,
- mitral valve disease.

The Criteria Committee of the New York Heart Association (1994) classification of heart failure is often used to assess the severity of the condition (see Box 3.1). This classification is divided into four classes ranging from patients who have few symptoms to patients who are unable to carry out the activities of daily living. Although acute LVF is not included in this classification, the classification system offers useful background understanding to the concept of heart failure generally and the clinical features.

The underlying abnormality for the majority of patients with heart failure in the Western world is impaired left-ventricular systolic function secondary to ischaemic cardiomyopathy (Cowie et al., 2000). The New York Heart Association (NYHA) classification ranges from class I – no symptoms, although left-ventricular systolic impairment is evident on echocardiogram – to class IV – severe symptoms of breathlessness at rest (Criteria Committee of the New York Heart Association, 1994). Despite maximal drug

---

**Box 3.1 The New York Heart Association (NYHA) scale for classification of heart failure**

**NYHA I** Patients have no limitation on activities and experience no symptoms from ordinary activities; however, there is evidence of left-ventricular impairment on echocardiography.

**NYHA II** Patients experience mild limitation of activity; they are comfortable at rest or with mild exertion. Evidence of mild to moderate left-ventricular impairment on echocardiography.

**NYHA III** Patients experience marked limitation of activity; they are comfortable only at rest. Evidence of moderate to severe left-ventricular impairment on echocardiography.

**NYHA IV** Patients confined to bed or chair; even minimal activity causes discomfort and symptoms occur at rest. Evidence of severe left-ventricular impairment on echocardiography.

Source: Criteria Committee of the New York Heart Association (1994).

---

treatment with angiotensin-converting enzyme (ACE) inhibitors, diuretics and beta-blockers, many patients still experience symptoms of breathlessness on minimal exertion or rest (NYHA classes III and IV). This limitation has a marked impact on quality of life (NICE, 2003). Patients with these symptoms will probably experience recurrent and prolonged hospital admissions for episodes of decompensation (acute episodes of worsening symptoms) because of failure of the heart to compensate for the disease and increased loss of independence; indeed, the management would focus upon the self-management of symptoms.

### Pathogenesis
When the heart begins to fail, compensatory neurohormonal activity begins that activates the sympathetic nervous system and the renin–angiotensin–aldosterone system. The sympathetic

nervous system is activated by impulses sent to baroreceptors and chemoreceptors located mainly in the aortic arch and the carotid sinus (Albert, 1999).

- Baroreceptors monitor blood pressure. When they detect a fall in blood pressure due to heart failure they stimulate the cardiovascular centre in the brain, which stimulates the sino-atrial node to increase the heart rate.
- Chemoreceptors detect chemical changes, such as a lack of oxygen, which causes the sympathetic nervous system to release noradrenaline (norepinephrine) and adrenaline (epinephrine), and results in vasoconstriction, which increases blood pressure.

The renin–angiotensin–aldosterone system is activated when there is a decrease in kidney perfusion. Renin acts on angiotensin (a liver substrate) to produce angiotensin I, which passes through the lungs and is converted to angiotensin II. This is a vasoconstrictor, which causes an increase in blood pressure and the release of aldosterone, which promotes the re-absorption of sodium and water (Jackson et al., 2000). Antidiuretic hormone is also activated, which causes vasoconstriction (Piano et al., 1998) and the retention of sodium and water. Peripheral resistance is increased, which eventually increases cardiac output but only for a short time. With the increase in blood volume the heart has to work harder to pump the blood around the body, which impairs heart function even further. Pulmonary oedema is often a presenting sign, as the acute leeching out of fluid into the interstitial spaces over a short period of time is a dramatic (and frightening for the patient) feature of LVF. See dyspnoea below.

Death is most commonly due to ventricular arrhythmia or progressive pump failure. Studies report a mortality of close to 40% within 1 year of diagnosis and around 10% each year thereafter. However, some earlier studies, such as the Hillingdon Heart Study were carried out before the widespread introduction of beta-blockers and specialist heart-failure nurses (Cowie et al., 1999, 2000). Echocardiography, cardiac catheterisation and nuclear medicine have since improved the diagnosis and investigation of patients with heart failure.

### Clinical features

Clinical features include

- anxiety,
- tachycardia,
- dyspnoea,
- fatigue,
- pallor,
- hypotension,
- diaphoresis (sweating),
- cool extremities at rest.

The triad of hypotension (systolic blood pressure <90 mmHg), oliguria and low cardiac output constitutes a diagnosis of cardiogenic shock (see p. 95).

Severe acute heart failure and cardiogenic shock may be related to an extensive MI, sustained cardiac arrhythmias (for example, atrial fibrillation or ventricular tachycardia) or mechanical problems (for example, acute papillary muscle rupture or post-infarction ventricular septal defect).

#### *Dyspnoea (shortness of breath) on exertion*

The first symptom most patients experience is breathlessness. When the left ventricle fails to eject sufficient volumes of blood into the systemic circulation there is an increase in left-ventricular end-diastolic pressure (LVEDP), an increase of which means that there will be an elevation of pressure in the pulmonary vasculature and this may lead to pulmonary oedema with tachycardia (Piano et al., 1998). This can be acutely worrying for the patient and may be the reason for their presentation.

#### *Orthopnoea and paroxysmal nocturnal dyspnoea*

Nocturnal dyspnoea ('cardiac asthma'; shortness of breath that occurs hours or minutes after lying down) is another symptom of heart failure. When a patient lies down there is an increase in left-ventricular filling pressures because of the increase in venous return from the peripheral extremities. Congestion of blood in the heart results in an increase in systemic venous pressure leading to widespread oedema (Addison and Thomas, 1998).

## Oedema

Oedema is an excessive accumulation of fluid in the interstitial spaces of the tissues. Rapid onset of pulmonary oedema is a dramatic feature of LVF, as outlined above. Patients with right-sided heart failure, sometimes known as CHF, can develop systemic oedema, which ranges from mild ankle oedema to gross oedema of the legs, abdomen, sacrum and scrotum (Addison and Thomas, 1998; Watson et al., 2000).

## Confusion and memory impairment

In severe heart failure, patients may not be able to sleep because of shortness of breath and anxiety. Disturbance in sleep patterns and reduced blood flow to the brain may also cause confusion (Watson et al., 2000).

## Treatment

When patients are admitted to hospital with heart failure it is important that they are assessed and their main problems identified and their care planned. Acute and chronic management strategies in heart failure are aimed at improving both symptoms and prognosis, although management in individual patients will depend on the underlying aetiology and the severity of the condition. It is imperative that the diagnosis of heart failure is accompanied by an urgent attempt to establish its cause, as timely intervention may greatly improve the prognosis (Millane et al., 2000).

The aims of treatment are to:

- reduce the symptoms of dyspnoea (most important),
- reduce cardiac filling pressures,

- reduce vascular resistance,
- increase cardiac output,
- reduce excess intravascular volume (be aware that these patients may be intravascularly volume depleted secondary to chronic diuretic use).

Milestone 2 of Chapter 6 of the National Service Framework for Coronary Heart Disease (Department of Health, 2000) asserts that every hospital should have an agreed protocol for the management of suspected and confirmed heart failure.

The priorities of care, initially, are as follows.

- Assess the patient following the ABCDE approach (Chapter 1). Evaluate MEWS score and alert medics/outreach if necessary (see p. 298).
- Ensure that the patient has a clear airway – if the patient has an altered conscious level, their airway is at risk.
- Sit the patient in an upright position and administer high-flow oxygen using a non-rebreathe mask (see Figure 1.4). Establish oxygen saturation monitoring using a pulse oximeter; the patient should be monitored in a high-dependency area.
- Insert a wide-bore intravenous (IV) cannula (e.g. 14 gauge).
- Establish continuous ECG monitoring: arrhythmias are common and can be life-threatening (Resuscitation Council UK, 2006).
- Monitor the patient's vital signs closely with frequent re-assessments: deterioration may be rapid; include blood pressure, temperature, pulse, respiratory rate, fluid balance, blood glucose, arterial blood gases and urea and electrolytes.
- Correction of hypoperfusion will correct the metabolic acidosis; consider inserting a central venous catheter to monitor central venous pressure (e.g. in critical illness).
- Consider cautious use of IV loop diuretics, such as frusemide (furosemide), induce transient venodilatation, when administered to patients with pulmonary oedema, and this may lead to symptomatic improvement even before the onset of diuresis.
- Cautious use of IV opiates or opioids (morphine or diamorphine) are an important adjunct in the management of severe

acute heart failure, by relieving anxiety, pain and distress, and reducing myocardial oxygen demand. They also produce transient venodilatation, thus reducing preload, cardiac filling pressures and pulmonary congestion (Millane et al., 2000). Be aware that they may cause respiratory depression.

- Nitrates (sublingual, buccal and IV) may also reduce preload and cardiac filling pressures and are particularly valuable in patients with both angina and heart failure.
- In cases of severe refractory heart failure in which the cardiac output remains critically low, the circulation can be supported for a critical period of time with inotropic agents. For example, dobutamine and dopamine (or Levosimenden) have positive inotropic actions, acting on the $\beta_1$-receptors in cardiac muscle (Jackson et al., 2000).
- Consider insertion of a urinary catheter to closely monitor urine output.
- Involve the heart-failure team at the earliest opportunity (Department of Health, 2000). Appropriate specialist on-going care is essential.
- Consider balloon-pump and non-invasive ventilation involving CPAP or BiPAP (see Chapter 2) in a specialist environment.

In summary, a basic overview has been presented of the concept of heart failure, in an attempt to offer greater understanding of the emergency nature of acute LVF – this is a sudden cardiac emergency that is particularly distressing and frightening for the patient and carer – its aetiology can be both cardiac and non-cardiac. A good understanding with a systematic application of assessment and care is essential in reducing the risk of this potentially life-threatening cardiac event. Alerting medical staff immediately to this situation, and ensuring the most appropriate evidence-based treatment strategies are applied, is essential.

## ACUTE CORONARY SYNDROMES

The term acute coronary syndrome (ACS) defines a spectrum of clinical presentations of the same disease process; from unstable angina (ischaemic pain without myocardial damage, including new-onset angina), through non-ST-segment elevation MI (NSTEMI), to ST-segment-elevation myocardial infarction (STEMI). ACS should be distinguished from stable angina, which develops during exertion and resolves at rest. In contrast, unstable angina occurs suddenly, often at rest or with minimal exertion, or at lesser degrees of exertion than the individual's previous angina.

Many cardiac arrests are caused by underlying coronary artery disease and occur in the context of an ACS (Resuscitation Council UK, 2006). It is therefore essential that practitioners understand the basis of ACS and implement appropriate treatment strategies. This is guided initially be the patient's symptoms and ECG changes. Treatment should not be delayed to await the appearance of biochemical markers that may not be detectable for several hours after the onset of symptoms (Edwards & Pitcher, 2005). It is worth noting that 50% of high risk ACSs will have a possible Troponin at presentation. The aim for all patients is universal: to alleviate symptoms, resuscitate if necessary and provide prompt and effective restoration or protection of coronary blood flow to relieve ischaemia and prevent further myocardial damage. Ultimately this will reduce the risk of cardiac arrest and death.

## Pathogenesis

The common underlying causative mechanism is sudden fissuring, erosion or rupture of the cap of an atherosclerotic plaque in a coronary artery. Subendothelial collagen becomes exposed and promotes platelet adhesion, aggregation and activation. A surrounding fibrin-rich thrombus develops around the platelets and is accompanied by a complex set of reactions including vasoconstriction, inflammation and micro-embolism (Edwards & Pitcher, 2005). The result is reduced coronary arterial blood flow but the pathological and clinical consequences are variable depending upon whether occlusion of the coronary artery is partial or total; on the degree of collateral blood flow to the affected myocardium; and on the mass of myocardium affected (Figure 3.1).

## Clinical features

Clinical features of ACS include:

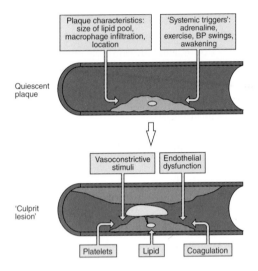

**Figure 3.1** Unstable plaque 'culprit lesion'

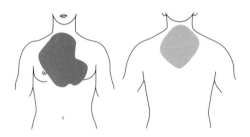

**Figure 3.2** The typical distribution of chest pain in ACS, front and back

- chest pain (Figure 3.2),
  - characteristic, excruciating, 'crushing', 'throbbing' type of pain, retrosternal, radiates to the left shoulder, left ulnar part of arm, lower jaw, neck, abdomen to the umbilicus,
  - lasts for a longer time than anginal pain, usually >30 min,
  - may have its onset at rest, unlike stable angina,
  - not relieved by rest or nitroglycerine,

○ 15–20% of infarcts are painless, especially in diabetes mellitus and in the elderly: in these cases it may present as acute onset of breathlessness and signs of pulmonary oedema;
- shortness of breath;
- nausea;
- vomiting;
- diaphoresis (sweating);
- palpitations;
- anxiety or sense of impending doom;
- a feeling of being acutely ill.

### Diagnosis

ACS is only one of the many potential causes of chest pain; however, it is safer to treat the patient as if it is cardiac in origin until proven otherwise.

Initial examination will include;

- reported history of acute cardiac ischaemia,
  ○ abrupt new onset of severe ischaemic chest pain, deterioration of previously stable angina or crescendo anginal symptoms in frequency and severity;
- 12-lead ECG;
- blood tests (in particular serum cardiac markers such as troponin I/T and/or creatine kinase (CK)-MB (Table 3.1), but also

**Table 3.1** Cardiac markers in response to myocardial injury

| Serum marker of myocardial injury | Detected (h) | Peak (h) | Falls | Normal value ($\mu$g/l) |
|---|---|---|---|---|
| Myoglobin | 1–3 | 1–8 | 12–18 h | <1 |
| CK-MB isoforms | 1–6 | 4–8 | 12–48 h | <1 |
| Troponin complex | 3–6 | 10–24 | Troponin I: 5–9 days<br>Troponin T: 7–14 days | <0.4<br><0.01<br>>0.1<br>(indicative of an MI) |

including urea and electrolytes, random glucose, random cholesterol and full blood count);
- chest X-ray (portable; only if the cause is not thought to be cardiac; it is not appropriate to send the patient to the X-ray department in the acute situation).

Results from these tests will be evaluated in conjunction with a rapid history and examination focusing primarily on the cardio-vascular system (Connaughton, 2001).

### Basic ECG monitoring and recording considerations

*Preparing the skin*: remove any chest hair with a disposable razor and dry the skin if sweating or wet.

*Obtaining good contact with skin and electrodes*: slight abrasion of the skin before electrode placement to remove dry skin will improve the conduction signal. Apply slight pressure to ensure good contact between electrode gel and skin.

*Placing the electrodes* (Figure 3.3): place an electrode on each arm and leg, avoiding large muscle mass. Chest lead positions:

- $V_1$ fourth intercostal space right of the sternum,
- $V_2$ fourth intercostal space left of the sternum,

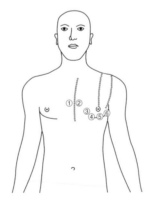

**Figure 3.3** Placement of the electrodes when undertaking a 12-lead ECG

- $V_3$ midway between $V_2$ and $V_4$,
- $V_4$ fifth intercostal space midclavicular line,
- $V_5$ fifth intercostal space in line with the anterior axillary line,
- $V_6$ fifth intercostal space mid-axilla.

*Eliminating muscle tremor and artifact*: Placing the limb electrodes on bone rather than muscle can help to eliminate muscle tremor. Encourage the patient to stay still and relax to obtain a good-quality trace. Maintain the patient's dignity by covering the chest with a light blanket or sheet. Colour-coding of leads is universal to help the operator ensure that lead-connection errors are minimised. Always make sure you have placed the leads in the correct position. Common mistakes are made with the limb leads, which can be mixed up.

The ECG leads consist of:

- limb leads: I, II, III, aVR, $aV_L$, $aV_F$;
- inferior leads: II, III, $aV_F$;
- lateral leads: I, aVL;
- precordial or chest leads: $V_1$–$V_6$, generally called the anterior leads but can be separated into right ventricle ($V_1$, $V_2$), ventricular septum ($V_3$, $V_4$) and anterolateral left ventricle ($V_5$, $V_6$).

The ST-elevation changes in the various ECG leads can be attributed to occlusion of specific arteries or infarct-related artery (IRA) as follows:

- inferior MI represents occlusion of the right coronary artery;
- anterior MI represents occlusion of the left coronary artery (main stem) or left anterior descending artery;
- lateral MI represents occlusion of the circumflex coronary artery (Table 3.2 and Figure 3.8).

### Cardiac enzymes

As ACS is now recognised as a single clinical entity which represents the entire clinical spectrum, the clinical approach focuses

**Table 3.2** ST-segment elevation and its relationship to the area of the heart affected

| MI region | Artery occluded | Leads showing ECG changes |
| --- | --- | --- |
| Anterior | LAD | $V_2$–$V_5$: 'anteroseptal chest leads' often I, $aV_L$ as well |
| Inferior | Right (usually) | II, III, $aV_F$ 'inferior leads' (record right-sided ECG – leads $V_{3R}$ and $V_{4R}$ are clinically significant) |
| Posterior | Right or circumflex | Difficult to see: posterior-wall infarction causes R wave (not Q wave) in $V_1$ with ST depression. Often associated with inferior MI (posterior 12-lead ECG is recommended: leads $V_7$–$V_9$ are clinically significant). |
| Lateral | Circumflex or diagonal branch of LAD | I, $aV_L$, $V_5$, $V_6$ 'lateral leads' |

LAD, left anterior descending.

upon risk stratification, to which cardiac markers have assumed a central role (Joint European Society of Cardiology/American College of Cardiology Committee, 2000; Fox et al., 2004) (see Table 3.3).

The best cardiac marker for each case depends on the time from onset of symptoms; the earliest markers are myoglobin and CK-MB isoforms (1–4 h). CK-MB and troponins are ideal in the intermediate period of 6–24 h. The troponins are recommended for elevation in patients who present more than 24 h after symptom onset.

The **CK-MB** fraction exists in two isoforms called 1 and 2, identified by electrophoretic methodology. The ratio of isoform 2 to 1 can provide information about myocardial injury. An isoform ratio of 1.7 or greater is considered an excellent indicator for early acute MI (Thompson, 2005). CK-MB isoform 2 demonstrates elevation even before CK-MB by laboratory testing. However, the disadvantage of this method is that it requires skilled labour because electrophoresis is required, and large numbers of samples

**Table 3.3** Spectrum of acute coronary syndrome

|  | **ACS with unstable angina** | **ACS with myocyte necrosis** | **ACS with clinical MI** |
|---|---|---|---|
| Marker | Tn and CK-MB undetectable | Tn elevated Tn T <1.0 ng/ml | Tn T >1.0 ng/ml ±↑CK-MB |
| ECG | ST↓ or T↓ Transient ST↑ Normal | ST↓ or T↓ Transient ST↑ Normal | ST↑ or ST↓ or T inversion May evolve Q waves |
| Risk of death | 5–8% | 8–12% | 12–15% |
| Pathology | Plaque disruption, intra-coronary thrombus, micro-emboli Partial coronary occlusion→complete coronary occlusion | | |
| LV function | No measurable dysfunction→systolic dysfunction, LV dilatation | | |

Source: adapted from Fox et al. (2004).
LV, left-ventricular; Tn, troponin.

cannot be run simultaneously or continuously. False-positive results with CHF and other conditions can occur. The release kinetics of the CK-MB isoforms is rapid. CK-MB2 is detected in serum 2–4 h after symptom onset and peaks at 6–9 h.

**Myoglobin** is an early marker of acute MI. It is a haem protein found in skeletal and cardiac muscle, its low molecular weight accounts for its early-release profile. Myoglobin typically rises 1–3 h after onset of infarction, peaks at 6–8 h and returns to normal within 24–36 h (Newby et al., 2001).

Cardiac troponins are regulatory proteins of the thin actin filaments of the cardiac muscle. **Troponin T** and **troponin I** are highly sensitive and specific markers of myocardial injury. Serial measurement of troponin I or troponin T has become an important tool for risk stratification of patients presenting with ACSs. The joint committee of the European Society of Cardiology, the American College of Cardiology and the American Heart Association (Braunwald et al., 2000) has recently accepted the measurement of troponin I and troponin T in serum as the standard biomarker for the diagnosis of acute MI and for diagnosis and management of ACSs.

However, cardiac troponins are not early markers of myocardial necrosis. They appear in serum within 3–6 h of symptom onset, similar in timing to the release of CK-MB; however, they remain elevated for as long as 24 days after an MI due to the gradual degeneration of myofibrils and release of troponin complex. An elevated troponin level enables risk stratification of patients with ACS and identifies patients at high risk of adverse cardiac events up to 6 months after the initial event (Lindahl et al., 1996). Indeed, there is a relationship between cardiac troponin levels and risk of death in patients with ACS (i.e. the greater the rise the greater the risk of death) (Fox et al., 2004; see Table 3.3).

Troponins have a number of advantages over other cardiac markers in specific clinical situations.

- Troponins are not normally present in serum unless cardiac cell necrosis has occurred. Thus, they are more cardiac-specific than CK-MB. This enhanced specificity allows for more accurate diagnosis of cardiac injury, especially in the presence of damage to skeletal muscle.
- Troponin levels remain elevated from 3 h and up to 24 days after MI. Thus, sensitivity remains high long after CK-MB and myoglobin levels have returned to normal. The increased sensitivity of troponins is an advantage in patients who delay seeking medical care for MI because of misleading symptoms.
- Studies evaluated the use of troponin T and troponin I as single prognostic indicators of mortality risk at the time of hospital admission. The results showed convincingly that elevated cardiac troponin levels are predictive of poor outcomes in patients with ACSs (Antman et al., 1996; Wu et al., 1994; Fox et al., 2004).

There are other non-cardiac conditions that troponins may be raised in (i.e. renal failure, heart failure, sepsis and acute pulmonary embolus); therefore, the clinical context is very important.

## Unstable angina

Unstable angina is defined by one or more of the following.

- Angina of effort occurring over a few days with increasing frequency provoked by progressively less exertion. This is commonly referred to as crescendo angina.
- Episodes of angina occurring recurrently and unpredictably, without specific provocation by exercise. These episodes may be relatively short-lived (e.g. a few minutes) and may settle spontaneously or be relieved temporarily by sublingual glyceryl trinitrate (GTN), before recurring within a few hours.
- An unprovoked and prolonged episode of chest pain, raising suspicion of acute MI, but without definite ECG or laboratory evidence of acute MI.
- New-onset angina is also considered unstable angina, since it suggests a new pathophysiologic process in the coronary artery.

In unstable angina, the ECG may

- be normal,
- show evidence of acute myocardial ischaemia (usually ST-segment depression), or
- show non-specific abnormalities (e.g. T-wave inversion) (see Figure 3.4).

In unstable angina, cardiac enzymes are usually normal, and troponin release is absent or very minor. Troponin release is a marker of increased risk and the level of risk increases with the level of troponin. ECG abnormality, especially ST-segment depression, is a marker of increased risk of further coronary events in patients with unstable angina. However, a normal ECG and absent troponin release do not necessarily mean that a patient with unstable angina is not at high risk of early further life-threatening coronary events. Only if the ECG and other markers of coronary risk (e.g. troponin) are normal, and further risk assessment (e.g. by exercise testing) does not indicate evidence of reversible myocardial ischaemia, should other possible causes

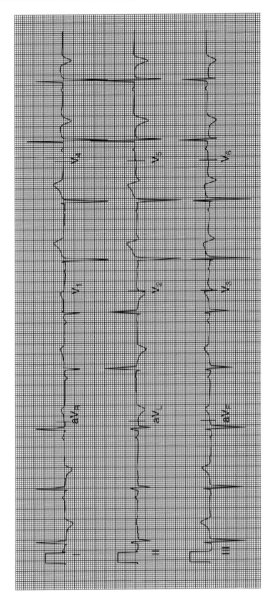

**Figure 3.4** ECG showing T-wave inversion significant in leads $V_2$–$V_6$

of acute chest pain be considered if the initial history suggested unstable angina (Connaughton, 2001).

### Non-ST-segment elevation MI (NSTEMI)

The diagnosis of NSTEMI is based upon a history of acute cardiac ischaemia in the absence of ST-segment elevation. In NSTEMI it is common for the ruptured atherosclerotic plaque to have caused incomplete coronary-artery occlusion. Alternatively, the myocardium may have been protected by good collateral flow or may have a relatively low oxygen demand. This different underlying situation is the basis for the differing effectiveness of and approaches to treatment from those used in ST-segment elevation MI (STEMI; see p. 76).

NSTEMI is characterised by the following:

- chest pain: felt as a heaviness, tightness or indigestion-like discomfort (may be in the upper abdomen) (see Figure 3.5);
- sustained chest pain for at least 20–30 min, often longer;
- pain may radiate into the throat, into one or both arms (more commonly the left), into the back or into the epigastrium

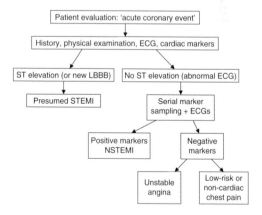

**Figure 3.5** Summary of the pathway of diagnosis within acute coronary syndrome
LBBB, left bundle branch block.

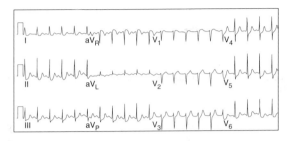

**Figure 3.6** 12-lead ECG demonstrating ST-segment depression in leads I, II, III, aV$_F$, V$_4$–V$_6$

(sometimes belching may be evident and this may be misinterpreted as evidence of indigestion);
- non-specific ECG changes: ST-segment depression/T-wave inversion (see Figure 3.6);
- raised troponin levels (the amount released reflects the extent of myocardial damage).

Treatment of NSTEMI and unstable angina are essentially the same and differ in some respect from the treatment of STEMI. Treatment is dictated largely by assessment of risk.

### Treatment of unstable angina and NSTEMI

If the ECG does not show ST-segment elevation, the term NSTEMI is applied. The accepted management of unstable angina and NSTEMI is empirical and initial treatment is guided by risk assessment. Patients are stratified, by haemodynamic, biochemical and medical factors, into high-, intermediate- and low-risk groups (European Society of Cardiology, 2002). It is risk status that drives pharmacological treatments and the timing of further interventional procedures (Antman et al., 2000) (thrombolysis in MI (TIMI) risk score; see Box 3.2).

Treatment for patients with unstable angina and NSTEMI typically consists of the following. First covered is the immediate period.

---

**Box 3.2 The TIMI (thrombolysis in MI) risk score for unstable angina/NSTEMI**

If present, each of the following contributes +1 to the overall score. A score >4 indicates high-risk non-ST-segment elevation ACS

- Age ≥65 years
- At least three risk factors for coronary artery disease: male sex, hyperlipidaemia, hypertension, smoking, diabetes mellitus, family history of premature coronary disease
- Previous coronary stenosis ≥50%
- ST-segment elevation or depression at presentation
- Two or more anginal events in the past 24 h
- Aspirin use in the past 7 days
- Elevated serum cardiac biomarkers

Source: Antman et al. (2000).

---

*Pain relief*

Effective pain relief is a priority and can be provided before a 12-lead ECG is recorded (Erhardt et al., 2002).

- Diamorphine is the preferred agent, administered intravenously and titrated according to response until all pain has dissipated.

*Anti-platelet agents*

Anti-platelet agents work on various steps of the platelet-aggregation pathway to prevent clot formation.

- Aspirin 300 mg (then 75–150 mg daily); should be administered early in all ACS unless absolutely contraindicated (ISIS 2, 1988);
- clopidogrel 300 mg (then 75 mg daily) (CURE Study Investigators, 2001; NICE, 2004);
- glycoprotein IIb/IIIa inhibitors are recommended as part of initial management of unstable angina or NSTEMI in those at high risk of MI or death (NICE, 2002a).

### Anti-thrombin agents

The use of heparin is recommended as an essential part of ACS treatment (Bertrand et al., 2002). Heparin blocks thrombin production, and can reduce thrombus formation and facilitate resolution.

- Low-molecular-weight heparin (e.g. enoxaparin 3–6 days) (ASSENT, 2002).

### Anti-ischaemic therapies

Anti-ischaemic therapies decrease myocardial oxygen use by decreasing heart rate, lowering blood pressure or decreasing left-ventricular contractility or inducing vasodilatation. They can also provide pain relief when ischaemia is the cause of pain (Erhardt et al., 2002).

- Nitrates (IV if high risk);
- beta-blockers (IV if high risk);
- calcium-channel blockers (for recurrent ischaemia, particularly if beta-blockers are contraindicated).

Once the patient's condition is stabilised, the focus of management shifts to preventing further cardiac events. This involves treatments to prevent future plaque rupture and thrombus formation. Control of blood pressure should be optimised and lipid-lowering therapy initiated.

The following medications have been shown to reduce the recurrence of cardiovascular events and should be used in secondary prevention regimens (Bertrand et al., 2002):

- Aspirin (75 mg/day);
- clopidogrel (75 mg/day for 12 months);
- angiotensin-converting enzyme (ACE) inhibitors;
- beta-blockers (bisoprolol 5 mg, atenolol 50 mg, metoprolol 50 mg);
- statins (3-hydroxy-3-methylglutaryl-CoA (HMG-CoA) reductase inhibitors).

- calcium antagonist (if beta-blockers are contraindicated);
- oral nitrate (imdur 30–60 mg, suscard buccal 2 or 5 mg).

These last two have been used for symptom relief.

Cardiac troponins are measured 12 h after onset of the pain (see p. 63). If this is positive, coronary angiography is typically performed on an urgent basis, as this is highly predictive of a heart attack in the near future. If the troponin is negative, a treadmill exercise test or a thallium scintigram may be requested (see Figure 3.7).

If any of the following risk factors are present, early angiography is indicated (Department of Health, 2000):

- elevated troponin T levels;
- prolonged rest angina with ECG changes in more than two leads;

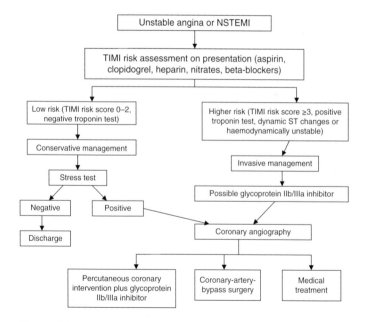

**Figure 3.7** A summary of the treatment for unstable angina and NSTEMI

- pulmonary oedema or hypotension;
- angina not settling with medical treatment;
- second presentation of ACS within 3 months;

### ST-segment elevation MI (STEMI)

Despite advances in primary and secondary treatments of ischaemic heart disease, approximately 240,000 patients per annum present with acute MI in England and Wales each year. The 30-day mortality remains around 50% and, of this group, 50% will die within the first 2 h (NICE, 2002b). It is well established that in some cases there is often a delay from the onset of symptoms to the patient calling for help; clearly this may be a contributing factor. In addition, an acute MI may cause ventricular fibrillation or asystole, one of the commonest causes of sudden cardiac arrest (Resuscitation Council UK, 2006). Many of these patients may die before ever reaching hospital.

The typical presentation of STEMI should be easily distinguishable to the emergency practitioner. The sudden development of crushing, retrosternal chest pain at rest, associated with sweating, nausea and sometimes light-headedness. The patient is often short of breath, appearing cold and clammy. Failure to triage such a patient to a high-dependency/resuscitation facility might be considered inexcusable (Thompson, 2005). Of course it must be remembered that not all patients with STEMI present in such a way. Any history of recent onset of chest or upper abdominal pain should alert the practitioner to rule out cardiac pain by assessing the patient more fully as a matter of priority; the triage category must represent the degree of urgency. The rapid undertaking of a 12-lead ECG is essential (see Table 3.2 and Figure 3.8).

### Priorities of care

The priorities for all ACSs are to:

- assess the patient in a high-dependency/resuscitation area following the ABCDE approach described in Chapter 1;

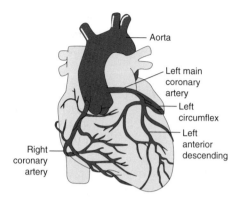

**Figure 3.8** A diagrammatical representation of the coronary arteries

- take the history and perform an examination focusing primarily on the cardiovascular system.

Examination may not reveal any obvious clinical findings, although it can be used to exclude non-cardiac causes of chest pain and identify non-ischaemic cardiac disorders, such as valve disease (Bertrand et al., 2002). Taking the patient's history involves the identification of risk factors for underlying coronary artery disease (Box 3.3). Identifying cardiac risk factors makes a diagnosis of ACS more likely, and may be particularly useful in patients with atypical symptoms (Coady, 2006).

- Sit the patient in a comfortable position and administer high-flow oxygen using a non-rebreathe mask (Figure 1.4). Establish oxygen-saturation monitoring using a pulse oximeter, aiming for a saturation of more than 95% (Booker, 2004).
- The patient should be monitored in a high-dependency area.
- Insert a wide-bore IV cannula (e.g. 14 gauge).
- Monitor the patient's vital signs closely with frequent re-assessments: deterioration may be rapid; include blood pressure, temperature, pulse and respiratory rate.
- Record the perceived severity of chest pain on an objective scale.

---

**Box 3.3 Risk factors for underlying coronary artery disease**

Aged over 65 years
Diabetes
Family history of coronary artery disease
Heart failure
Hyperlipidaemia
Hypertension
Male
Previous angina or myocardial infarction
Smoking

Sources: Fox (2004), Gibler et al. (2005).

---

Initial treatment for patients presenting with ACS can be memorised using the mnemonic MONA (Resuscitation Council UK, 2006):

- **M**orphine IV (e.g. diamorphine 2.5–5 mg; a total of 10–15 mg may be required to achieve pain relief, titrated to avoid sedation and respiratory depression) and anti-emetic (e.g. metoclopramide 10 mg);
- **O**xygen: continue high-flow oxygen therapy. There are few data on the specific benefits of oxygen use in this situation, but current guidelines advocate its routine use (Resuscitation Council UK, 2006). It is considered especially important if the $SaO_2$ is less than 90%, and is continued routinely for the first 2–3 h;
- **N**itroglycerin nitrate: sublingual GTN;
- **A**spirin 300 mg to chew, and then swallow, as soon as possible (NICE, 2007).

While initiating treatment according to MONA guidance, interpretation of the ECG is required to guide further management.

- Record a 12-lead ECG to guide further treatment based on definitive diagnosis, and establish continuous ECG monitoring: arrhythmias are common and life-threatening (Resuscitation Council UK, 2006).

- Consider clopidogrel (NICE, 2004, 2007).
- Take blood, via the IV line for
  - ○ urea and electrolytes,
  - ○ glucose,
  - ○ CK-MB, troponin or other serum cardiac markers,
  - ○ random cholesterol,
  - ○ full blood count.

These measures should take no longer than 10–15 min before proceeding to immediate treatment measures (Connaughton, 2001). If the ECG shows evidence of ST elevation, initial diagnosis of MI is highly likely and reperfusion should be considered immediately (Fibrinolytic Therapy Trialists' Collaborative Group, 1994; Boersma et al., 1996; Baigent et al., 1998); either primary PCI or thrombolytic therapy depending on local policy.

Although local guidelines may vary, common ECG criteria for thrombolysis are ST elevation of:

- 1 mm or more in two or more adjacent limb leads;
- 2 mm or more in two or more adjacent chest leads (Garcia & Holtz, 2001).

Or new left bundle branch block (LBBB).

*Pain management*

Pain management is a priority for the patient with ACS because pain increases myocardial oxygen demands (Woods et al., 2000). Interventions include opiate analgesics, oxygen therapy, nitrates and aspirin (NICE, 2007). Opiate analgesics are typically used to relieve acute cardiac pain. Despite this not all patients receive total pain relief; however, the sensation of pain is dulled and the patient feels more comfortable (Calvey & Williams, 1991). Opiates reduce the sensation of pain by affecting neurochemical transmission and thereby raising the patient's pain threshold. Although opiate analgesia has little direct affect on the causes of pain it does, however, have a number of positive indirect actions. This is achieved through the reduction of anxiety by reducing the adverse effects of adrenaline on the patient's heart rate. Reduction in heart rate reduces myocardial oxygen demand with an associated reduction in left-ventricular wall stress. An additional indirect benefit of opiates is the ability of opiates – primarily morphine and diamorphine – to produce vasodilation, and this has a positive effect on left-ventricular wall stress (Jowett & Thompson, 2003). Indeed, diamorphine (2.5–5 mg, depending on the severity) is the drug of choice and it is well tolerated following STEMI.

Opiates should be administered in conjunction with an anti-emetic to guard against opiate-induced nausea and vomiting, which may worsen the nausea typically associated with STEMI. Careful choice of anti-emetic agent is required as drugs like cyclizine may reduce the haemodynamic benefits of opiates (Jowett & Thompson, 2003) and therefore metoclopramide is the ideal initial agent.

Nitrates are well established in the management of ACS and can be quickly administered by sublingual, buccal routes or if required as a continuous IV infusion. They have the benefit of dealing directly with ischaemic pain as well as reducing cardiac workload (Gersh and Rahimtoola, 1997). The main effect of nitrates is not just their ability to dilate coronary arteries but their effect on myocardial oxygen demand. Nitrates reduce both preload and after load and this reduces cardiac workload and therefore myocardial oxygen demand (Opie, 1997; NICE, 2002b).

The effectiveness of re-assurance, patient information and looking after patients in a controlled environment by skilled practitioners is also an important aspect of pain relief and should not be under-estimated. The effectiveness of non-pharmacological interventions is difficult to measure; however, effective communication, calm mannerisms and involvement of relatives or life partners represents good care and is the cornerstone of non-pharmacological intervention (Castle, 2002).

*Reperfusion therapy*

The ECG is a crucial component of risk assessment and planning of treatment. Acute ST-segment elevation or new LBBB in a patient with a typical history of an acute coronary event is an indication for treatment through reperfusion therapy (see Table 3.2). Where primary PCI is available, then this is the preferred method and should occur within 90 minutes of diagnosis (see p. 93).

When the choice is thrombolytic drugs, it is the fibrinolytic system that is activated. Releasing plasminogen activators causes plasminogen to be deposited on fibrin strands in the thrombus. Plasminogen activators cleave plasminogen to release plasmin, which digests fibrin and fibrinogen, resulting in lysis of the clot. The aim is to recanalise the thrombolytic occlusion and restore blood flow (Rang et al., 2003). The optimum therapy aims to open the infarct-related artery as soon as possible. All patients with a relevant history and appropriate ECG should be given reperfusion therapy or have this option actively rejected. The National Service Framework guidelines clearly specify the importance of prompt provision of thrombolysis to relevant patients (Department of Health, 2000). Thrombolytic drugs reduce the mortality of patients with STEMI. If given early enough after onset of symptoms, they can reduce the severity of myocardial damage and represent the patient's best chance of survival. Although major clinical trials continue to determine the best strategies to be employed to further enhance the administration of thrombolytic therapy, one key factor is evident: the sooner thrombolysis is administered the better (Revell, 2000). There is overwhelming evidence of benefit from reperfusion therapy in patients presenting within 24 h of symptom onset (GISSI, 1986; ISIS 2, 1988; GISSI-2, 1990; ISIS 3, 1992; GUSTO, 1993). If the ECG confirms changes suggestive of STEMI (ST elevations in specific leads, a new LBBB or a true posterior MI pattern), thrombolytics may be administered or primary coronary angioplasty may be performed (Martini and Bartholomew, 2000).

Reperfusion therapies include the following.

*Thrombolytic agent*: the thrombolytic agent of choice is given intravenously and stimulates fibrinolysis, destroying blood clots obstructing the coronary arteries. The National Service Framework (Department of Health, 2000) expects 75% of eligible patients to receive thrombolysis within the 20-min target.

NICE (2002b) recommends that, in hospital, the choice of thrombolytic drug should take account of:

- the likely balance of benefit and harm (for example, stroke) to which each of the thrombolytic agents would expose the individual patient;
- current UK clinical practice, in which it is accepted that patients who have previously received streptokinase should not be treated with it again;
- the hospital's arrangements for reducing delays in the administration of thrombolysis.

Common thrombolytic agents include:

- streptokinase (infusion) – usually for cases of inferior MI;
- alteplase (bolus and infusion);
- tenecteplase (single bolus, weight adjusted, now replacing alteplase);
- reteplase (double bolus);
- heparin is given (usually intravenously) as a bolus prior to all thrombolytic drugs except streptokinase;
- in the pre-hospital settings bolus drugs (e.g. reteplase or tenecteplase) are recommended as the preferred option.

Ensuring the patient and his or her family are aware of the risks and benefits is vital to their making an informed decision. Although the risk of intracranial bleeding remains low at 0.5–1.4% (ISIS 3, 1992), an appropriately trained healthcare professional should discuss this factor with the patient (Humphreys & Smallwood, 2004).

There are certain criteria that must be assessed to deliver thrombolysis safely; these are divided into absolute and relative

---

**Box 3.4 Absolute and relative contraindications to thrombolysis**

**Absolute**
- Major surgery or trauma within 6 weeks
- Known allergy to planned agent
- Pregnancy
- Proven active peptic ulcer or bleed within 6 months
- Stroke within 6 months
- Intracranial tumours
- Bleeding disorder
- Aortic dissection

**Relative**
- Extensive cardiopulmonary resuscitation
- Severe hypertension
- Diabetic retinopathy

---

contraindications (Box 3.4). During administration of the therapy, the patient will require close observation for any complications, such as hypotension, allergic reaction, haemorrhage, arrhythmias and further chest pain (Thompson, 2005).

*Primary percutaneous coronary intervention (PCI)*: this option is becoming more popular as primary treatment for STEMI (Figure 3.9), particularly in the following cases:

- patients with a contraindication to thrombolysis,
- patients presenting with cardiogenic shock (see below),
- patients who re-infarct following thrombolysis,
- patients in whom thrombolysis fails (technically 'rescue' PCI),
- patients presenting to a centre where primary PCI is the preferred therapeutic modality (i.e. some tertiary centres; there are currently around 15 tertiary centres operating round-the-clock primary PCI services in the UK, 2008).

In this procedure, a flexible catheter is passed via the femoral or radial arteries and advanced to the heart to identify blockages in

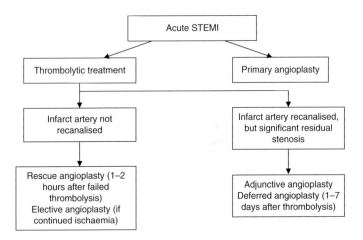

**Figure 3.9** A summary of the treatment choices for STEMI

the coronaries. When occlusions are found, they can be intervened upon mechanically with angioplasty and perhaps stent deployment if a lesion, termed the culprit lesion, is thought to be causing myocardial damage (Revell, 2000).

*Patient transfer*

It is important to remember that some high-risk patients may require urgent transfer to another hospital for percutaneous coronary intervention. This is likely to be a stressful period for patients and their families because they need to deal with the immediate health concern as well as travelling to an unfamiliar hospital which may be many miles from their home. Other issues such as work and finances can also heighten their anxiety. Nurses can minimise stress to patients and their families by co-ordinating the transfer and keeping the patient and family fully informed of arrangements. Supplying telephone numbers and contact names will help reduce some of these concerns.

Some nurses such as the ACS nurse may have specific responsibility for co-ordinating care and have a vital part to play if transfer to another hospital is needed (Coady, 2006). Responsibilities may include:

- assessing patients with ACS who are managed in a non-cardiac environment to ensure that they receive equitable care;
- liaising with the specialist care team following inter-hospital transfer for interventions, and keeping up to date with patients' progress and management;
- tracking patients as they move between departments, wards and hospitals;
- developing multi-professional ACS protocols including patient-transfer protocols that facilitate prompt transfer;
- educating other members of staff about ACS and its management.

In summary, early, prompt diagnosis and treatment are crucial life-saving interventions for the patient with ACS. Effective early pain relief remains a clinical priority as does patient re-assurance throughout the application of confident, skilful cardiac practice. The prompt referral of the patient to the appropriate specialist nursing team (ACS/Cardiac Assessment teams) at entry into hospital and the facilitation of timely care through patient-group directions (PGDs) will have a positive effect on the patient experience.

Chest pain has multiple causes that can be urgent and life-threatening or minor, requiring simple relief of pain and re-assurance. The nurse has a considerable role to play in ensuring that patients are assessed and cared for using effective evidence-based strategies; not only assisting the doctor in diagnosis but also alerting medical colleagues to high-risk patients.

## CARDIAC ARREST RHYTHMS

Cardiac arrhythmias can be sporadic and variable within medical cardiac emergencies. Interpretation of such arrhythmias, particularly those of cardiac arrest, plays an important role within the instigation of early, appropriate medical management. Early definitive treatment is essential to optimise chances of survival. In this section the arrhythmias of ventricular tachycardia (VT), ventricular fibrillation (VF), asystole and electromechanical dissociation (EMD) will be discussed, within the paradigms of shockable and non-shockable rhythms (Resuscitation Council UK, 2006) (see Figure 3.13).

### Shockable rhythms (VF/VT)

In adults, the commonest rhythm at the time of cardiac arrest is VF (Figure 3.10), which may be preceded by a period of VT (Figure 3.11), by a bradyarrhythmia or, less commonly, supraventricular tachycardia (SVT).

#### *Treatment of shockable rhythms (VF/VT)*

Having confirmed cardiac arrest, summon help (including a request for a defibrillator) and start cardiopulmonary resuscitation (CPR), beginning with chest compressions, with a compression/ventilation ratio of 30:2. As soon as the defibrillator arrives apply self-adhesive pads or paddles to the chest to diagnose the rhythm. If VF/VT is confirmed, follow the treatment steps below.

- Attempt defibrillation. Give one shock of 150–200 J biphasic (360 J monophasic); the exact joules to be given will be determined by your Trust guidelines: ensure that you are familiar with these.
- Immediately resume chest compressions (30:2) without re-assessing the rhythm or feeling for a pulse.
- Continue CPR for 2 min, then pause briefly to check the monitor.

If VF/VT persists:

- give a further (second) shock of 150–360 J biphasic (360 J monophasic),
- resume CPR immediately and continue for 2 min,
- pause briefly to check the monitor,
- if VF/VT persists give adrenaline 1 mg IV followed immediately by a (third) shock of 150–360 J biphasic (360 J monophasic),

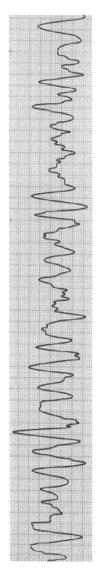

**Figure 3.10** Ventricular fibrillation (VF)

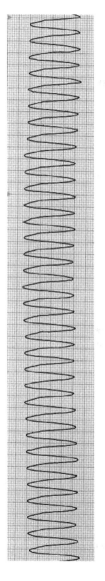

**Figure 3.11** Ventricular tachycardia (VT)

- resume CPR immediately and continue for 2 min,
- pause briefly to check the monitor,
- if VF/VT persists give amiodarone 300 mg IV followed immediately by a (fourth) shock of 150–360 J biphasic (360 J monophasic),
- resume CPR immediately and continue for 2 min,
- give adrenaline 1 mg IV immediately before alternate shocks (i.e., approximately every 3–5 min),
- give further shocks after each 2 min period of CPR and after confirming that VF/VT persists.

If organised electrical activity compatible with a cardiac output is seen, check for a pulse:

- if a pulse is present, start post-resuscitation care;
- if no pulse is present, continue CPR and switch to the non-shockable algorithm.

If asystole is seen, continue CPR and switch to the non-shockable algorithm.

### Non-shockable rhythms (pulseless electrical activity (PEA) and asystole)

Pulseless electrical activity (PEA) is defined as organised cardiac electrical activity in the absence of any palpable pulses: it can be any rhythm that one would normally expect to have an associated cardiac output. These patients often have some mechanical myocardial contractions but they are too weak to produce a detectable pulse or blood pressure. PEA may be caused by reversible conditions that can be treated. Survival following cardiac arrest with asystole or PEA is unlikely unless a reversible cause can be found and treated quickly and effectively.

*Treatment for PEA*

- Start CPR 30:2.
- Give adrenaline 1 mg IV as soon as IV access is achieved.

- Continue CPR 30:2 until the airway is secured, then continue chest compressions without pausing during ventilation.
- Recheck the rhythm after 2 min:
  - if organised electrical activity is seen, check for a pulse and/or signs of life:
    - if a pulse and/or signs of life are present, start post resuscitation care;
    - if no pulse and/or no signs of life are present (PEA):
      - continue CPR,
      - recheck the rhythm after 2 min and proceed accordingly,
      - give further adrenaline 1 mg IV every 3–5 min (alternate loops);
  - if there is VF/VT at rhythm check, change to shockable side of the algorithm;
  - if asystole or an agonal rhythm is seen at rhythm check:
    - continue CPR,
    - recheck the rhythm after 2 min and proceed accordingly,
    - give adrenaline 1 mg IV every 3–5 min (alternate loops).

*Treatment for asystole and slow PEA (rate <60 min)*

- Start CPR 30:2.
- Check that the leads are attached correctly without stopping CPR.
- Give adrenaline 1 mg IV as soon as IV access is achieved.
- Give atropine 3 mg IV (once only).
- Continue CPR 30:2 until the airway is secured, then continue chest compressions without pausing during ventilation.
- Recheck the rhythm after 2 min and proceed accordingly.
- If VF/VT recurs, change to the shockable rhythm algorithm.
- Give adrenaline 1 mg IV every 3–5 min (alternate loops).

**Asystole**

Asystole (Figure 3.12) is a condition that could be exacerbated or precipitated by excessive vagal discharge. This could be reversed by a drug that blocks the effect of vagal discharge. Therefore, give

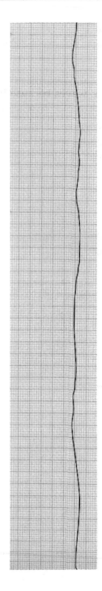

**Figure 3.12** Asystole

atropine 3 mg (the dose that will provide maximum vagal blockade) if there is asystole or the rhythm is slow PEA (rate <60 min).

Whenever a diagnosis of asystole is made, check the ECG carefully for the presence of P waves because in this situation ventricular standstill may be treated effectively by cardiac pacing. Attempts to pace true asystole are unlikely to be successful (Resuscitation Council UK, 2006). Treatment options are summarised within the Adult Advance Life Support algorithm (Figure 3.13).

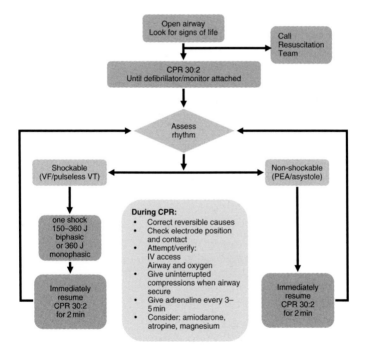

**Figure 3.13** The Adult Advanced Life Support algorithm (Resuscitation Council UK, 2006)

**Reversible causes**

Potential causes or aggravating factors for which specific treatment exists must be considered during any cardiac arrest. For ease of memory, these are divided into two groups of four, based upon their initial letter: either H or T (Resuscitation Council UK, 2006):

- **H**ypoxia,
- **H**ypovolaemia,
- **H**yperkalaemia, hypokalaemia, hypoglycaemia, hypocalcaemia, acidaemia and other metabolic disorders,
- **H**ypothermia,
- **T**ension pneumothorax,
- **T**amponade,
- **T**oxins,
- **T**hrombosis (pulmonary embolism or coronary thrombosis).

**Cardiac tamponade**

The pericardial cavity is a potential space between the parietal and visceral layers of the pericardium. This cavity normally contains between 30 and 50 ml of serous fluid that acts as a lubricant as the heart contracts and relaxes. This volume can increase to 1 litre in some chronic conditions, such as progressive malignant pericardial effusion with compromising pericardium. If fluid builds up gradually, the pericardium can stretch to contain as much as 1 litre of fluid without affecting the heart (Porth, 1994). However, if it accumulates rapidly, even an increase as little as 50 ml can exert enough pressure on the heart to be life-threatening (Humphreys, 2006). Indeed, cardiac tamponade is considered to be a life-threatening event.

*Pathogenesis*

As the fluid accumulates within the pericardial sac, the diastolic pressure in each chamber rises so that filling the chambers is impaired (Lilly, 1998, Thompson, 2005). The increase of systemic venous pressure results in signs of right-sided heart failure:

distension of the jugular veins, oedema and hepatomegaly. Decreased atrial filling leads to inadequate ventricular filling; reduced cardiac output and potential circulatory collapse (Tortora and Anagnostakos, 2000). Pulsus paradoxus, in which arterial blood pressure during expiration exceeds arterial pressure during inspiration by more than 10 mmHg, is a key indicator of cardiac tamponade. Normally, inspiration has little effect on cardiac flow or volume. In addition, reduced filling of the ventricles during diastole decreases blood availability for systolic stroke volume, and cardiac output declines. Failure to decompress the heart leads to inadequate perfusion of vital organs, shock and ultimately death (Resuscitation Council UK, 2006).

### Signs and symptoms of cardiac tamponade

Cardiac tamponade should be suspected in any patient with known pericarditis, pericardial effusion or chest trauma who develops signs and symptoms of systemic vascular congestion and decreased cardiac output (Humphreys, 2006). Key physical findings include:

- jugular venous distension,
- systemic hypotension,
- a small, quiet heart on physical examination (muffled heart sounds), due to the insulating effects of effusion (McCance and Huether, 1998).

These three are known as Beck's triade.

Other signs include:

- sinus tachycardia and pulsus paradoxus,
- dyspnoea and tachypnoea, which reflect pulmonary congestion, as well as decreased oxygen delivery to peripheral tissues.

Acute haemorrhage into the pericardium is also a result of left-ventricular free-wall rupture following MI, and frequently presents as chest pain, haemodynamic collapse and PEA (Connaughton, 2001). This occurs in between 1 and 4% of people post-MI and is usually rapidly fatal; in this instance the patient will present in cardiac arrest. During a cardiac arrest, cardiac tamponade is difficult to diagnose because the typical signs of distended neck veins and hypotension cannot be assessed. However, cardiac arrest after penetrating chest trauma should raise strong suspicions of tamponade (Dracup, 1995).

*Treatment*

The priorities initially are as follows.

- Assess the patient following the ABCDE approach (Chapter 1). Evaluate MEWS score and alert medics/outreach if necessary (see p. 298).
- If the patient has altered conscious level then the airway is at risk – summon urgent medical help – this is a rapidly deteriorating life-threatening event.
- Administer high-flow oxygen using a non-rebreathe mask (Figure 1.4). Establish monitoring of oxygen saturation using a pulse oximeter.
- Ensure that patient has a wide-bore IV cannula in place (e.g. 14 gauge).
- Establish continuous ECG monitoring; consider undertaking a 12-lead ECG. If tamponade has developed slowly over weeks or months, the ECG will share the characteristics of a pericardial effusion (Humphreys, 2006). In acute emergency situations, it is inappropriate to record a 12-lead ECG because immediate resuscitation and the removal of high-pressure pericardial fluid using pericardiocentesis or resuscitative thoracotomy are the only measures that can reverse this life-threatening condition (Resuscitation Council UK, 2006).
- Monitor the patient's vital signs closely with frequent re-assessments: deterioration may be rapid; include blood pressure, temperature, pulse and respiratory rate.
- Prepare for immediate pericardiocentesis (undertaken by medical staff).

In summary, cardiac tamponade is a life-threatening event. Astute observations for the signs and symptoms of cardiac tamponade are critical to expedite treatment for this potentially life-threaten-ing complication (Humphreys, 2006; Resuscitation Council UK, 2006).

## Cardiogenic shock

Cardiogenic shock is characterised as LVF of the heart itself, which results in reduced tissue perfusion and impaired cellular activity (De Jong, 1997). It can result from heart failure of any cause (McCance and Huether, 1998), and it leads to the heart ceasing to function as an effective pump. Although most cases tend to follow an acute MI, particularly anterior-wall infarcts, other causes include cardiomyopathies, tamponade, arrhythmias, valve disease, pericardial infection and heart failure resulting from drug toxicity (Nolan et al., 1998). Cardiogenic shock is more common in older patients, those with diabetes, females and patients with a history of MI, usually developing within 24 h of admission to hospital. In 85% of cases it is attributable to exten-sive anterior infarct and in only 15% of patients is it because of potentially reversible complications. This is one of the reasons why prognosis is poor, with an in-hospital mortality rate of 80% or more (Nolan et al., 1998).

### Pathogenesis

Due to the state of low cardiac output, there is a reduction in arterial blood pressure. The baroreceptors then release both nor-adrenaline and adrenaline, hormones that cause an increase in the contractility of the heart and also cause vasoconstriction within the body. Due to the damage to the heart muscle, the increase in heart rate will probably do little to increase cardiac output. This tachycardia can also be detrimental to the heart, as it is being placed under more pressure and requires a greater oxygen supply to the heart muscle that is already ischaemic due to the shock (Collins, 2000). The falling cardiac output and blood pressure cause poor perfusion of blood to the tissues and eventu-ally the cells are unable to maintain cellular homoeostasis. The resultant hypoxia causes widespread vasodilation due to lactic acidosis, resulting in a further drop in blood pressure that the compensatory mechanisms are unable to prevent. Pulmonary oedema will eventually occur when the pulmonary circulation and the right side of the heart also begin to fail. Despite recent advances in haemodynamic monitoring and drug therapy, the mortality rate remains high, with 80% of patients dying from cardiogenic shock (Alexander et al., 1994).

### Signs and symptoms of cardiogenic shock

The signs and symptoms are caused by the widespread impairment of cellular metabolism. They include:

- fast, weak pulse,
- falling blood pressure (systolic pressure <90 mmHg),
- cold clammy skin,
- oliguria (or falling urine output, <30 ml/h),
- dyspnoea (from pulmonary oedema),
- confusion (due to poor cerebral perfusion),
- nausea and vomiting,
- associated chest pain and arrhythmias (Nolan et al., 1998).

### Treatment

The priorities initially are as follows.

- Assess the patient following the ABCDE approach (Chapter 1). Evaluate MEWS score and alert medics/outreach if necessary (see p. 298).
- If the patient is having severe breathing difficulties, his airway is at risk – summon urgent medical help.
- Sit the patient in an upright position and administer high flow oxygen using a non-rebreathe mask (Figure 1.4). Establish monitoring of oxygen saturation using a pulse oximeter; this may be difficult due to peripheral circulatory shut-down.
- Ensure that the patient has a wide bore IV cannula in place (e.g. 14 gauge).
- Establish continuous ECG monitoring: arrhythmias are common and can be life-threatening (Resuscitation Council UK, 2006), undertake a 12-lead ECG.

- Monitor the patient's vital signs closely with frequent re-assessments: deterioration may be rapid; include blood pressure, temperature, pulse, respiratory rate (particularly rate and depth) and fluid balance.
- Urine output needs hourly accurate measurement: a catheter will need to be inserted (Hand, 2001).
- Blood investigations include glucose, arterial blood gases, urea and electrolytes and cardiac enzymes if indicated.
- Control of pain and anxiety are important at this stage:
  - IV morphine is often administered as it also dilates blood vessels, and reducing peripheral resistance. Morphine might help to relieve anxiety, which is vital as patients usually find the condition distressing.
- Medication is an important aspect of treating cardiogenic shock.
  - High doses of diuretics are often used to reduce excess fluid. This reduces the pressure that the heart has to work against, and to treat pulmonary oedema (Sheppard & Wright, 2000). Loop diuretics, such as frusemide, are only effective because of their mild vasodilatory action, rather than their diuretic action. This vasodilation reduces what is known as preload: the amount of blood returning to the heart. If this is reduced, the heart does not have to pump as hard to empty its chambers, so reducing congestion. If vasodilation creates further capacity for the increased blood volume, then specific vasodilatory drugs are also important.
  - Sublingual GTN spray might create widespread vasodilation, thus resolving the symptoms (Sheppard & Wright, 2000).
  - Inotropes will enhance the patients' haemodynamic state: IV dobutamine (5–20 μg/kg per min) is the usual choice of drug given via a peripheral line, along with dopamine (2.5–5.0 μg/kg per min) via a central line to improve renal blood flow.
  - Patients may need to be transferred to a high-dependency area (intensive care unit) where an infusion of noradrenaline

(adrenaline may also be considered) could be considered and more invasive haemodynamic monitoring (such as arterial catheterisation) is available (Garretson, 2005). Balloon pumping may also be considered, which is usually managed within the coronary care unit.

In summary, cardiogenic shock is a life-threatening condition arising from a failure of the body to maintain cellular homoeostasis, resulting in cardiovascular collapse. It is a medical emergency and it is essential that practitioners are able to identify and treat patients in cardiogenic shock. Regular assessment and accurate monitoring of patients most at risk of cardiogenic shock is crucial to ensure early and timely critical intervention.

## REFERENCES

Addison, C & Thomas, K (1998) Heart failure. In Shuldham C (ed.), *Cardiorespiratory Nursing*. Stanley Thornes, Cheltenham

Albert, N (1999) Heart failure: the physiologic basis for current therapeutic concepts. *Critical Care Nurse* **19**(3), 2–13

Alexander, M, Fawcett, J & Runciman, P (1994) *Nursing Practice. The Adult*. Churchill Livingstone, Singapore

Antman, EM, Tanasijevic, MJ & Thompson, B (1996) Cardiac-specific troponin I levels to predict the risk of mortality in patients with acute coronary syndromes. *New England Journal of Medicine* **335**(18), 1342–9

Antman, E, Cohen, M, Bernink, P & McCabe, CH (2000) The TIMI risk score for unstable angina/non-ST elevation MI: a method for prognostication and therapeutic decision making. *Journal of the American Medical Association* **284**(7), 835–42

ASSENT (2002) The Assessment of the Safety and Efficacy of a New Thrombolytic Regimen (ASSENT)-3 Investigators. Efficacy and safety of tenecteplase in combination with enoxaparin, abciximab, or unfractionated heparin: the ASSENT-3 randomized trial in acute myocardial infarction. *Lancet* **358**, 605–13

Baigent, C, Collins, R, Appleby, P & Parish, S (1998) ISIS-2: 10-year survival among patients with suspected acute myocardial infarction in randomised comparison of intravenous streptokinase, oral aspirin, both, or neither. The ISIS-2 (Second International Study of Infarct Survival) Collaborative Group. *British Medical Journal* **316**(7141), 1337–43

Bertrand, ME, Simoons, ML & Fox, KA (2002) Management of acute coronary syndromes in patients presenting without persistent ST-segment elevation. *European Heart Journal* **23**(23), 1809–40

Boersma, E, Maas, AC, Deckers, JW & Simoons, ML (1996) Early thrombolytic treatment in acute myocardial infarction: reappraisal of the golden hour. *Lancet* **348**(9030), 771–5

Booker, R (2004) The effective assessment of acute breathlessness in a patient. *Nursing Times* **100**(24), 61

Braunwald, E, Antman, EM, Beasley, JW, Califf, RM, Cheitlin, MD & Hochman, JS (2000) ACC/AHA guidelines for the management of patients with unstable angina and non-ST-segment elevation myocardial infarction: executive summary and recommendations. A report of the American College of Cardiology/American Heart Association task force on practice guidelines (committee on the management of patients with unstable angina). *Circulation* **102**, 1193–1209

British Heart Foundation (2004) Coronary Heart Disease Statistics Database. *www.heartstats.org* (accessed 21 February 2005). British Heart Foundation, London

Calvey, T & Williams, N (1991) *Principles and Practice of Pharmacology for Anaesthetists*, 2nd edn. Blackwell Scientific Publications, London

Castle, N (2002) Acute coronary syndromes. *Emergency Nurse* **10**(2), 19–22

Coady, E (2006) Managing patients with non-ST-segment elevation acute coronary syndrome. *Nursing Standard* **20**(37), 49–56

Collins, T (2000) Understanding shock. *Nursing Standard* **14**(49), 35–9

Connaughton, M (2001) *Evidence-Based Coronary Care.* Churchill Livingstone, London

Cowie, MR, Wood, DA, Coats, AJ, Thompson, SG, Poole-Wilson, PA & Suresh, V (1999) Incidence and aetiology of heart failure: a population-based study. *European Heart Journal* **20**(6), 421–8

Cowie, MR, Wood, DA & Coats, AJ (2000) Survival of patients with new diagnosis of heart failure: a population based study. *Heart* **83**(5), 505–10

Criteria Committee of the New York Heart Association (CCNYHA) (1994) *Nomenclature and Criteria for Diagnosis of Diseases of the Heart and Great Vessels*, 9th edn. Little, Brown & Co, Boston, MA

CURE Study Investigators (2001) Effects of clopidogrel in addition to aspirin in patients with acute coronary syndromes without ST-segment elevation. *New England Journal of Medicine* **345**, 494–502

De Jong, MJ (1997) Clinical snapshot: cardiogenic shock. *American Journal of Nursing* **97**(6), 40–1

Department of Health (2000) *National Service Framework for Coronary Heart Disease. Modern Standard and Service Models.* Department of Health, London

Dracup, K (1995) *Meltzer's Intensive Coronary Care: a Manual for Nurses*, 5th edn. Prentice Hall International (UK), London

Edwards, N & Pitcher, D (2005) An overview of acute coronary syndromes. *British Journal of Resuscitation* **4**(1), 6–10

Erhardt, L, Herlitz, J & Bossaert, L (2002) Task force on the management of chest pain. *European Heart Journal* **23**(15), 1153–76

European Society of Cardiology. The Task Force on the Management of Acute Coronary Syndromes (2002) Management of acute coronary syndromes in patients presenting without persistent ST segment elevation (ESC). *European Heart Journal* **23**, 1809–40

Fibrinolytic Therapy Trialists' Collaborative Group (1994) Indications for fibrinolytic therapy in suspected acute myocardial infarction: collaborative overview of early mortality and major morbidity results from all randomised trials of more than 1000 patients. *Lancet* **343**(8893), 311–22

Fox, KA (2004) Management of acute coronary syndromes: an update. *Heart* **90**(6), 698–706

Fox, KA, Birkhead, J, Wilcox, C, Knight, C & Barth, J (2004) British Cardiac Society Working Group on the definition of myocardial infarction. *Heart* **90**(6), 603–9

Garcia, TB & Holtz, NE (2001) *Introduction to 12-lead ECG: the art of interpretation*. Jones and Bartlett Publishers, London

Garretson, S (2005) Haemodynamic monitoring: arterial catheters. *Nursing Standard* **19**(31), 55–64

Gersh, B & Rahimtoola, S (1997) *Acute Myocardial Infarction; Current Topics in Cardiology*, 2nd edn. Chapman and Hill, New York

Gibler, WB, Cannon, CP & Blomkalns, AL (2005) Practical implementation of the guidelines for unstable angina/ non-ST-segment elevation myocardial infarction in the emergency department: a scientific statement from the American Heart Association Council on Clinical Cardiology (Subcommittee on Acute Cardiac Care), Council on Cardiovascular Nursing, and Quality of Care and Outcomes Research Interdisciplinary Working Group, in Collaboration With the Society of Chest Pain Centers. *Circulation* **111**(20), 2699–710

Global Utilisation of Streptokinase & Tissue Plasminogen Activator for Occluded Coronary Arteries. The GUSTO Investigators (1993) An international randomised trial comparing 4 thrombolytic strategies for acute myocardial infarction. *New England Journal of Medicine* **329**, 673–82

Gruppo Italiano per lo Studio della Streptochinasi nell'Infarcto Miocardico (GISSI) (1986) Effectiveness of intravenous thrombolytic therapy in acute myocardial infarction. *Lancet* **1**, 397–401

Gruppo Italiano per lo Studio della Streptochinasi nell'Infarcto Miocardico (GISSI-2) (1990) A factorial randomised trial of alteplase versus streptokinase and heparin versus no heparin among 12490 patients with acute myocardial infarction. *Lancet* **336**, 65–71

Hand, H (2001) Shock. *Nursing Standard* **15**(48), 45–52

Humphreys, M (2006) Pericardial conditions: signs, symptoms and electrocardiogram changes. *Emergency Nurse* **14**(1), 30–6

Humphreys, M & Smallwood, A (2004) An exploration of the ethical dimensions pertinent to gaining consent for thrombolysis. *Nursing in Critical Care* **9**(6), 264–70

ISIS 2 (1988) Second international study of infarct survival collaborative group. A randomized trial of intravenous streptokinase, oral aspirin, both or neither among 17,187 cases of suspected acute myocardial infarction. *Lancet* **2**, 349–60

ISIS 3 (1992) Third international study of infarct survival collaborative group. A randomized comparison of streptokinase verses tissue plasinogen activator verses ansistreplase and aspirin plus heparin verses alone among 41,299 cases of suspected acute myocardial infarction. *Lancet* **339**, 753–70

Jackson, G, Gibbs, G, Davies, MK & Lip, GYH (2000) ABC of heart failure pathophysiology. *British Medical Journal* **320**(7228), 167–70

Joint European Society of Cardiology/American College of Cardiology Committee (2000) Myocardial infarction redefined: a consensus document of the Joint European Society of Cardiology/American College of Cardiology committee for the redefinition of myocardial infarction. *European Heart Journal* **21**, 1502–13

Jowett, N & Thompson, D (2003) *Comprehensive Coronary Care*, 3rd edn. Scutari Press, London

Lilly, LS (1998) *Pathophysiology of Heart Disease: a Collaborative Project of Medical Students and Faculty*, 2nd edn. Lea & Febiger, London

Lindahl, B, Venge, P & Wallentin, L (1996) Relation between troponin T and the risk of subsequent cardiac events in unstable coronary artery disease. The FRISC study group. *Circulation* **93**(9), 1651–7

Martini, F & Bartholomew, MS (2000) *Essentials of Anatomy and Physiology*, 2nd edn. Prentice Hall, London

McCance, KL & Huether, SE (1998) *Pathophysiology: the Biologic Basis for Disease in Adults and Children*, 3rd edn. Mosby Year Book, St Louis, MO

Millane, T, Jackson, G, Gibbs, CR & Lip, GYH (2000) ABC of heart failure. Acute and chronic management strategies. *British Medical Journal* **320**(7228), 559–62

Neubauer, S (2007). The failing heart – an engine out of fuel. *New England Journal of Medicine* **356**(11), 1140–51

Newby, LK, Storrow, AB & Gibler, WB (2001) Bedside multi-marker testing for risk stratification in chest pain units: the chest pain evaluation by creatine kinase- MB, myoglobin, and troponin I (CHECKMATE) study. *Circulation* **103**(14), 1832

NICE (2002a) *Technology Appraisal Guidance 47. Glycoprotein IIb/IIIa Inhibitor Guidance for Acute Coronary Syndromes.* NICE, London

NICE (2002b) *Technology Appraisal Guidance 52. Guidance on the Use of Drugs for Early thrombolysis in the Treatment of Acute Myocardial Infarction.* NICE, London

NICE (2003) *Technology Appraisal Guidance 5. Chronic Heart Failure. Management of Chronic Heart Failure in Adults in Primary and Secondary Care.* Clinical Guideline 5. NICE, London

NICE (2004) *Technology Appraisal Guidance 80. Clopidogrel in the Treatment of Non-ST Segment-elevation Acute Coronary Syndrome.* NICE, London

NICE (2007) *Clinical Guideline 4, MI: secondary prevention.* NICE, London (replaces NICE inherited guideline A, 2001)

Nolan, J, Greenwood, J & MacKintosh, A (1998) *Cardiac Emergencies: a Pocket Guide.* Butterworth Heinemann, Oxford

Opie, L (1997) *Drugs for the Heart*, 4th edn. WB Saunders and Co, Philadelphia, PA

Piano, M, Bondmass, DW & Schwetz, DW (1998) The molecular and cellular pathophysiology of heart failure. *Heart and Lung: The Journal of Critical Care* **27**(1), 3–19

Porth, CM (1994) *Pathophysiology: Concepts of Altered Health States*, 4th edn. Lippincott, Philadelphia, PA

Rang, H, Dale, MM, Ritter, JM & Moore, PK (2003) *Pharmacology.* Churchill Livingstone, Edinburgh

Resuscitation Council UK (2006) *Advanced Life Support Provider Manual*, 5th edn. Resuscitation Council UK, London

Revell, D (2000) Thrombolytic therapy: an A&E perspective. *Emergency Nurse* **8**(8), 32–8

Sheppard, M & Wright, M (2000) *Principles and Practice of High Dependency Nursing*. Baillière Tindall, London

Thompson, PL (2005) *Coronary Care Manual*, 2nd edn. Churchill Livingstone: London

Tortora, GJ & Anagnostakos, NP (2000) *Principles of Anatomy and Physiology*, 7th edn. Harper Collins, New York

Unal, B, Critchley, JA & Capewell, S (2004) Explaining the decline in coronary heart disease mortality in England and Wales 1981–2000. *Circulation* **109**(9), 1101–7

Watson, R, Gibbs, CR & Lip, GYH (2000) ABC of heart failure: clinical features and complications. *British Medical Journal* **320**(7229), 236–9

Woods, S, Froelicher, E & Motzer, S (2000) *Cardiac Nursing*, 4th edn. Lippincott Williams & Wilkins, Philadelphia, PA

Wu, AH, Valdes, R & Apple, FS (1994) Cardiac troponin-T immunoassay for diagnosis of acute myocardial infarction. *Clinical Chemistry* **40**(6), 900–7

# Cardiovascular Emergencies

## Melanie Humphreys

**4**

## INTRODUCTION
Cardiovascular emergencies are life-threatening disorders that must be assessed and diagnosed quickly to avoid a delay in treatment and to minimise morbidity and mortality. Activity, levels of anxiety, speed of onset and previous experience may influence patients' perception of the significance of their illness. Through a structured approach of assessment, initiating investigations, treatment and delivering appropriate care, potential life-threatening cardiovascular events can be identified, alerting medical/surgical staff immediately to these situations, and ensuring that the most appropriate evidence-based treatment strategies are adopted.

The aim of this chapter is to allow the reader to understand the treatment of cardiovascular emergencies.

## LEARNING OUTCOMES
At the end of this chapter the reader will be able to:

❏ discuss the treatment of deep-vein thrombosis (DVT),
❏ discuss the treatment of pulmonary embolism,
❏ outline the treatment of sickle cell crisis,
❏ describe the treatment of hypertensive crisis,
❏ discuss the treatment of dissecting abdominal and thoracic aneurysms.

## DEEP-VEIN THROMBOSIS (DVT)
DVT is the single most preventable thrombo-embolic disorder, and is asymptomatic in many cases. It usually begins when small

deposits of fibrin collect in the deep veins of the thigh or calf as a result of slow blood flow and local activation of the clotting cascade. DVT can be asymptomatic, but the classic symptoms of calf pain, swelling, increased skin temperature, superficial venous dilation and (occasionally) pitting oedema usually occur when a thrombus becomes large enough to cause blood outflow problems (Gorman et al., 2000). Complete occlusion of a vein is rare, but can lead to a cyanotic discoloration of the limb and severe oedema, which can develop into venous gangrene (Kumar & Clark, 2002). DVT can resolve completely without causing patients any ill effects, but its prevention and treatment are important, since it can lead to a fatal pulmonary embolism.

More than 25,000 patients in England die each year from venous thrombo-embolism (VTE), which is more than the combined total of deaths from breast cancer, acquired immune deficiency syndrome (AIDS) and road traffic injuries (House of Commons Health Committee, 2005). Many of these deaths are preventable. By recognising high-risk patients, and starting them on what is proven to be a safe and cost-effective prophylactic treatment, lives can be saved.

**Pathogenesis**

Venous thrombosis is a condition in which a blood clot (thrombus) forms in a vein. This manifests clinically as a DVT, commonly in the deep veins of the legs, thighs and pelvis; and is a pulmonary embolism if the clot breaks off from the site in which it was created and lodges in the lung vessels (Robinson, 2006). DVT and pulmonary embolism are collectively known as venous thrombo-embolism (VTE). Thrombus formation is a result of an imbalance between the anti-coagulant and pro-coagulant systems in the blood (Enders et al., 2002). Three pathological processes, known collectively as Virchow's triad, have been shown to promote this imbalance and predispose to VTE formation (Wallis & Autar, 2001; United Kingdom Venous Thromboembolism Registry, 2004).

**Virchow's Triad**

1 *Venous trauma*: trauma or damage to vascular endothelium as a result of infection can lead to the release of tissue factor, which initiates the clotting cascade, leading to clot formation.
2 *Venous stasis*: vessel compression by enlarged lymph nodes, bulky tumours or previous thromboses can lead to venous stasis, as can immobility or confinement to bed; this is one of the main reasons why hospital inpatients are at increased risk of VTE.
3 *Hypercoagulability*: genetic conditions such as thrombophilia, which affects one in 20 of the UK population and causes the blood to clot more easily than it should, increase the chances of thrombus formation. Cancers, particularly adenocarcinomas and metastatic cancers, and oestrogens, found in oral contraceptives and hormone-replacement therapy, can also activate the clotting system, increasing the risk of VTE.

(Enders *et al.*, 2002; Turpie *et al.*, 2002; House of Commons Health Committee, 2005)

Clot formation is a complex process in which fibrinogen, a soluble protein in blood, is converted to a fibrin clot by the action of thrombin. This process is important in reducing blood loss when vessels are damaged or ruptured. Injury to vessel walls exposes collagen and releases tissue factor, a protein expressed by cell surfaces. This leads to a complex cascade of reactions in which various coagulation factors activate one another. Although this process is important in the repair of damaged vessels, the clotting cascade can be initiated in high-risk patients, resulting in thrombus formation and causing symptoms of VTE (Kumar & Clark, 2002).

**Risk factors**

Surgery and acute myocardial infarction (MI) are well-recognised major risk factors for VTE and, as a consequence, these groups of patients are provided routinely with prophylaxis (Anderson & Spencer, 2003). General medical patients are also at risk.

Factors that promote venous stasis, hypercoagulability or vascular damage contribute to the risk of VTE. The more risk factors a person has, the greater their risk of developing VTE. Prophylaxis in hospitalised patients is extremely important because they often have multiple risk factors (Welch, 2006).

**Signs and symptoms**

There are up to six signs and symptoms that might demonstrate a DVT episode. However, it should be acknowledged that in up to 50% of cases there are few or no significant physical abnormalities or clinical signs to be detected (Wallis & Autar, 2001). If signs are present, any resolution of the DVT might be demonstrated by a reduction in signs and symptoms.

*Abnormal swelling of the affected limb*

This can be due to localised oedema resulting from:

- thrombosis occlusion of the affected deep vein, which impedes venous blood return and can also affect the efficiency of collateral venous drainage;
- capillary damage, causing leakage of intravascular fluid into the surrounding tissues (extravasation), distal to the thrombosis site. Some departments still advocate bilateral baseline limb-girth measurements to be performed daily (Wallis & Autar, 2001); however, practitioners need to be aware of the potential for inter-operator variation. Furthermore, the absence of a significant difference between the limbs does not exclude a DVT.

*Warmth of affected limb*

In some cases, the affected limb feels warm to the touch. This might be due to localised venous congestion and accumulation of tissue metabolites in the affected limb (Kumar & Clark, 2002).

*Localised pain*

Lower-limb pain might be experienced in the calf muscle region during dorsiflexion movements of the foot: this is referred to as a positive Homans' sign. Although a number of reports have questioned the clinical utility of Homans' sign, it is often still used in clinical practice (Urbano, 2001).

Localised symptoms are commonly due to oedema in the tissues surrounding the site of thrombophlebitis (inflammation of vein where clot is present). Pain is not always present, for example, in cases where there is a small-sized thrombus with few localised inflammatory activities (Welch, 2006). However, in cases of iliofemoral vein thrombosis, extreme pain can present (Kumar & Clark, 2002).

### Dilation of veins

Due to the venous thrombus occlusion of the respective vein, a distal dilatation of veins might occur as a result of systemic and peripheral venous circulatory-stasis obstruction (Tortora & Anagnostakos, 2000).

### Colour changes of the leg

Initially, as a result of the venous thrombosis, pallor of the leg might be the only indicator. In other cases, a peripheral skin erythema (redness) of the affected limb occurs immediately over the DVT site, which might be due to the superficial thrombophlebitis (Hinchliff, 1996).

### Pyrexia

A systemic increase in body temperature to 39–40°C can be caused by the accumulation of tissue metabolites at the site of the thrombosis formation, and intravascular thrombophlebitis occurs (Brooker, 1998; Marieb, 1998).

### Asymptomatic

In 50% of cases the DVT has no initial observable symptoms and, of patients with a pulmonary embolism, up to 75% might have no sign of a preceding DVT (Kumar & Clark, 2002). As it is estimated that only one in nine cases will present clinically, all patients who are identified to be at risk should be assessed carefully, examined and monitored (Welch, 2006).

### Diagnosis

A diagnosis of DVT based solely on the evaluation of clinical signs has proven unreliable, and a combination of specific diagnostic procedures should be performed (Urbano, 2001), to direct management.

- Clinical risk stratification.
- D-dimer blood test (see Box 4.1).
- Ultrasound Doppler testing: this measures venous flow by placing a Doppler probe over veins, and the procedure can be performed with the patient standing. This test is useful for differentiating between a DVT and muscle strain or haematoma (Lewis & Collier, 1992).
- Ultrasonography: ultrasound is not 100% reliable, and those patients who are clinically suspected of having a DVT but have a negative ultrasound result should ideally have the test repeated a week later (Turpie et al., 2002).
- Contrast venography: this can detect a thrombus using a radio-opaque intravenous (IV) injection technique via the dorsal foot vein. It is suggested that many below-knee thrombi can be detected only by venography (Kumar & Clark, 2002).

---

**Box 4.1 The D-dimer blood test**

D-dimers are protein derivatives of fibrin found in plasma and produced when fibrin is degraded by plasmin (also known as fibrin-degradation products). Plasma concentrations of D-dimers are therefore raised in patients with venous thromboembolism (VTE). A positive diagnosis of VTE cannot be made using a D-dimer blood test alone, since levels can also be raised during infection, malignancy and pregnancy, and after an operation. D-dimers have a high negative predictive value, so if a patient with suspected VTE has a normal D-dimer blood test, the diagnosis can be ruled out. D-dimer testing is not indicated in patients with a high clinical probability of pulmonary embolism, since the test is almost certainly going to be positive and adds little to the clinical picture (Tovey & Wyatt, 2003).

---

## Treatment

Research supports the advantages of early anti-coagulation programmes following medical assessment and diagnosis of DVT, reducing the risk of pulmonary embolism to less than 1% (Levine et al., 1996). It must be acknowledged that whereas a clinical improvement of DVT does occur, the achievement of a complete clot breakdown via the natural fibrinolytic system occurs at a very low rate, as anti-coagulants have no pharmacological action in lysing existing thrombi (Urbano, 2001).

DVT and non-massive pulmonary embolism (see below) are treated similarly:

- low-molecular-weight heparin (LMWH),
- oral anti-coagulation (warfarin is the most widely used oral anti-coagulant).

Heparin therapy promotes the action of antithrombin and Factor III, which inhibits Factors X and XI in anti-coagulant doses. It also slows the clotting time by inhibition of prothrombin–thrombin, and further prevents conversion of fibrinogen to fibrin (Brooker, 1998).

In conjunction with heparin, oral anti-coagulant therapy is initiated, using warfarin as a first-choice anti-coagulant. Phenindione, an oral anti-coagulant should be used if the patient is allergic to warfarin (British National Formulary, 2005). Warfarin inhibits the vitamin K-dependent clotting factors and some naturally occurring proteins (particularly C- and S-anti-coagulants). Warfarin therapy should be overlapped with heparin therapy for 4–5 days as the anti-coagulant effects take at least 48–72 h to develop fully. Initial therapeutic doses, such as 10 mg warfarin per day, might be given for 2 days and the subsequent maintenance dose varies between patients and depends on the prothrombin time, which is reported universally as the international normalised ratio (INR).

For DVT patients receiving anti-coagulant therapy, an INR in the range 2.5–3.0 is desirable unless the patient has experienced a recent thrombosis. Treatment is usually maintained for approximately 3–6 months (British National Formulary, 2005; Welch, 2006).

### Anti-embolism stockings

In line with evidence-based nursing practice, anti-embolism stockings are used widely in the UK for all low-risk patients and are combined with other prophylaxis for moderate- and high-risk groups. Graduated compression stockings are designed to achieve a pressure gradient, with pressure increasing from the ankle to the thigh. The sequential compression profile of the stocking is aimed to mimic the deep leg-vein calf-muscle pumps, to promote efficient and effective emptying of vein circuits and respective valvular systems without adverse effects on arterial circulation (Wallis & Autar, 2001).

Healthcare practitioners have a vital role to ensure efficacy and safe wearing of the anti-embolism stockings. It is necessary to include localised physical assessment of the lower limbs and systemic assessment of the patient's health status. Accurate measurement and safe fitting of the stockings is of paramount importance to achieve optimum prophylaxis and patient compliance (Welch, 2006).

Anti-embolism stockings are frequently available in knee-length, thigh-length and special thigh-length with waistbelt versions, and might be colour-coded to distinguish between different types and sizes. Below-knee stockings are used for patients whose thigh circumference measures more than 84 cm, and for specific orthopaedic surgical procedures where the patient is to have wound incision above the popliteal joint, such as a femoral prosthesis or total hip replacement. Full-length stockings should be fitted in all other cases to achieve protection of the femoral vein. They must not be rolled down as this can cause a tourniquet effect in the femoral circulation and can predispose to a localised DVT. To encourage safe use and optimum patient compliance, it is important to demonstrate the correct fitting technique of the stocking. This should be supported by a follow-up discussion session, to elicit the do's and don't when wearing the stocking. Fitting guides on individual patient assessment, practical fitting, wearability and maintenance are supplied with the stockings, and practitioners should always refer to the manufacturer's literature when measuring and fitting patients for anti-embolism stockings (Wallis & Autar, 2001).

## PULMONARY EMBOLISM

A pulmonary embolism is an obstruction of part of the pulmonary vascular tree, usually caused by a thrombus that has travelled from a distant site; for example, the deep veins in the leg. The annual incidence is 60–70 per 100,000; it is a common cause of breathlessness and pleuritic pain (Robinson, 2006). Postmortem studies estimate that 10% of hospital deaths can be attributed to pulmonary embolism; 70% of these occur in medical patients and three-quarters are unrecognised before post-mortem (Gerotziafas & Samama, 2004).

Pulmonary embolism has an untreated mortality rate of about 30% and is the commonest cause of death after elective surgery, accounting for up to 15% of all post-operative deaths (Kakkar & De Lorenzo, 1998). It is the commonest cause of maternal death in the UK (McColl et al., 1997). Most thrombi are generated in the deep venous system of the lower leg and pelvis. Venous stasis is increased by immobility and dehydration, which leads to the accumulation of clotting factors and platelets. Up to 50% of leg thrombi embolise; clots above the knee do so more commonly than clots below the knee. Large clots may lodge at the bifurcation of the main pulmonary arteries, causing haemodynamic compromise. Smaller clots travel more distally, infarcting the lung and causing pleuritic pain (Robinson, 2006).

### Signs and symptoms

- Breathlessness and tachypnoea,
- pleuritic chest pain,
- occasionally haemoptysis.

In the instance of a massive pulmonary embolism, leading to cardiac arrest:

- collapse,
- hypotension,
- hypoxia,
- may show signs of engorged neck veins,
- right-ventricular gallop (a loud, additional heart rhythm).

**Diagnosis**

Patients with suspected pulmonary embolism should have initial routine investigations including:

- chest X-ray, ECG and arterial blood gases (to exclude other causes);
- a D-dimer blood test (see Box 4.1), a negative result, can reliably exclude diagnosis in patients considered of low probability for pulmonary embolism, and further imaging is not required in such patients.

Patients with a high clinical probability of pulmonary embolism (that is, multiple risk factors and ECG changes suggestive of pulmonary embolism), and those with low to intermediate probability but with a positive D-dimer blood test, should have further investigations.

- Isotope lung scanning (commonly known as a ventilation/perfusion or V/Q scan) is usually the initial investigation to be implemented. This may be unreliable in patients with chronic cardiac or respiratory disease.
- In these cases of chronic cardiac or respiratory disease, patients go on to have a computed tomographic pulmonary angiography (CTPA), which is quicker to perform, rarely needs to be followed by other imaging and may provide the correct diagnosis if pulmonary embolism is excluded.
- Since 70% of patients with proven pulmonary embolism have proximal DVT, ultrasound scanning of the legs has also been

suggested as the initial imaging test to confirm VTE (British Thoracic Society Standards of Care Committee, 2003).

A clinically massive pulmonary embolism can be diagnosed reliably with CTPA and echocardiography. Such imaging should be performed within 1 h of presentation; imaging should be within 24 h in cases of non-massive pulmonary embolism (British Thoracic Society Standards of Care Committee, 2003).

The majority of pulmonary embolisms are re-absorbed spontaneously and cause no ill effects once treated: anti-coagulation therapy for patients with non-massive pulmonary embolism is the same as described above for treatment of DVT. The altered blood flow and impaired gas exchange caused by a massive pulmonary embolism, however, result in decreased pulmonary compliance or even pulmonary infarction, leading to haemodynamic compromise, which can be fatal. Patients who survive may have increased pulmonary vascular resistance, which can lead to pulmonary hypertension and heart failure (Enders et al., 2002).

**Treatment**

For this group of patients the priorities initially are as follows.

- Assess the patient following the ABCDE approach (Chapter 1). Evaluate MEWS score and alert medics/outreach if necessary (see p. 298).
- Administer high flow oxygen using a non-rebreathe mask (see Figure 1.4). Establish monitoring of oxygen saturation using a pulse oximeter.
- Ensure that the patient has a wide-bore IV cannula in place (e.g. 14 gauge).
- If the patient has had a massive pulmonary embolism (where cardiac arrest is imminent, summon urgent medical help) thrombolysis with a bolus of 50 mg alteplase is recommended, although this should not be used as a first-line treatment in non-massive pulmonary embolism (British Thoracic Society Standards of Care Committee, 2003).
- Establish continuous ECG monitoring and undertake a 12-lead ECG.

- Monitor the patient's vital signs closely with frequent re-assessments: deterioration may be rapid; include blood pressure, temperature, pulse and respiratory rate.
- Prepare for transfer to high-dependency care area.

In summary, VTE is a potentially fatal condition that needs to be recognised and treated appropriately. DVT may display no significant physical abnormalities or clinical signs, and detection can prove difficult, it is the nurse's role to inform, teach and advise patients in relation to anti-coagulant medications, physiotherapy exercises and the practical wearability of anti-embolism stockings. Pulmonary embolism has the potential to be life-threatening, so astute observations for the signs and symptoms are critical to expedite efficient and effective treatment.

## SICKLE CELL CRISIS

A sickle cell disorder is a blood condition that is associated with the inheritance of sickle haemoglobin. The disorder affects haemoglobin, the red blood pigment responsible for carrying oxygen around the body, causing the blood cells to change shape or 'sickle'. Sickle haemoglobin is more prevalent in people of African and African-Caribbean origin, but is also found in other groups such as those with origins in the Mediterranean or the Indian subcontinent (Modell, 2005). A Birmingham study also identified babies from the white indigenous population who were sickle cell carriers (Eboh, 1996). It is estimated that in England there are more than 12,500 people with sickle cell disorders and 240,000 healthy carriers of the sickle gene variant. About 300 babies are born each year with sickle cell disorders and more than one in every 2400 births in England is affected by sickle cell disorders (Streetly, 2004).

### Pathogenesis

Sickle cell disease (SCD) is a chronic haemolytic anaemia characterised by the production of sickle haemoglobin (HbS). HbS is formed by a single point mutation of the amino acid structure on the surface of the molecule. Valine is substituted for glutamic acid in the sixth position of the beta-globin chain, causing insolubility of HbS in its deoxygenated state (Mehta & Hoffbrand, 2000). Deoxy-haemoglobin S forms rigid polymers, and subsequently causes cells to assume a sickle shape. These may return to their normal shape on reoxygenation; however, after repeated sickling episodes the erythrocytes become irreversibly sickled cells. Compared with healthy erythrocytes, sickled cells are not very flexible and have difficulty passing through small capillaries. Occlusion causes localised tissue hypoxia, in turn promoting further sickling. This blockage of vessels, lack of oxygen and subsequent tissue necrosis accounts for most of the clinical features of SCD (McKenzie, 1996).

*Three types of crisis that can occur in SCD*

- Vaso-occlusive crisis is the commonest and is also known as the painful crisis. As described above, sickled cells block capillaries and pain is caused by infarction. This can occur in the bones or any of the organs, and pain can be localised or diffuse. Vaso-occlusive crisis can occur spontaneously, lasts from days to weeks, and also tends to subside spontaneously (Bennett, 2005).
- Visceral sequestration crisis is characterised by pooling of red blood cells in the liver, spleen or lungs caused by sickling, and, although less common, can be fatal.
- Aplastic crisis can occur following infection by B19 parvovirus. This causes a temporary pause in the production of red blood cells, precipitating a severe acute-on-chronic anaemia (Mehta & Hoffbrand, 2000).

Factors known to trigger a crisis include infection, dehydration, acidosis, hypoxia, exercise, cold, altitude, pregnancy, alcohol and stress.

**Signs and symptoms of sickle cell crisis**

Most SCD sufferers experience a 'prodromal' stage, where a gradual build-up of symptoms can occur for days before a crisis, although more commonly the warning signs are present for less than an hour beforehand (Murray & May, 1988). During a crisis, patients may present with a condition known as chest syndrome. This is associated with:

- difficulty in breathing,
- pulmonary oedema,
- pyrexia,
- cough and anaemia,
- chest pain may or may not always be present.

The aetiology of chest syndrome is not clear, but it can occur as a result of infarction, visceral sequestration, infection or pulmonary fat embolism. The incidence is more common in adults, and it accounts for the highest cause of death in SCD patients (McKenzie, 1996).

Similarly, abdominal pain during a crisis is often referred to as girdle syndrome and can be caused by visceral sequestration in the mesenteric or hepatic circulation. The pain associated with the abdominal crisis of SCD is constant and sudden. It becomes unrelenting. The pain may or may not be localized to any one area of the abdomen. Nausea, vomiting and diarrhoea may or may not occur.

Joint crisis may also occur, and may develop without a significant traumatic history. Its focus is either in a single joint or in multiple joints. Often the connecting bony parts of the joint are painful. Range of motion is often restricted because of the pain.

Other symptoms experienced by patients with SCD, due to acute or chronic tissue infarction, include:

- avascular necrosis of the femoral and humeral heads or other bones,
- thrombosis, such as strokes,
- recurrent priapism,
- chronic or spontaneous leg ulcers,
- cardiomyopathy and other cardiac complications,
- retinopathy and hearing loss,

- painful swelling and deformity of the hands and feet in children called hand-foot syndrome or Dactylitis,
- renal papillary necrosis leading to urinary symptoms.

(Mehta & Hoffbrand, 2000; Newcombe, 2002)

### Treatment

The management of people with sickle cell disorders involves treating pain episodes and complications, understanding the seriousness of infections (and their potential to lead to a crisis) and addressing the psychological, social and cultural needs of patients: the potential for repeated admissions in a critical condition will necessitate the instigation of on-going support from the multidisciplinary team (Claster & Vichinsky, 2003). Patients with SCD presenting at the emergency department with a crisis should be triaged in the very urgent category; this means anyone with known SCD and experiencing severe pain should be seen by a doctor within 10 min of arrival in the department.

The priorities initially are as follows.

- Assess the patient following the ABCDE approach (Chapter 1). Evaluate MEWS score and alert medics/outreach if necessary (see p. 298).
- Administer high-flow oxygen using a non-rebreathe mask (Figure 1.4). Establish monitoring of oxygen saturation using a pulse oximeter.
- Ensure that the patient has a wide-bore IV cannula in place (e.g. 14 gauge). This may need to be undertaken by an expert. Remember the cannulation can be difficult in the SCD patient. Administration of IV fluids.
- Monitor the patient's vital signs closely with frequent reassessments: deterioration may be rapid; include blood pressure, temperature, pulse and respiratory rate.
- Following the initial assessment, the administration of an appropriate opiate analgesic (morphine or diamorphine) should precede any further assessment: it is likely that the

patient will be unable to co-operate with a full clinical examination initially and the movement involved may also exacerbate the pain (Maxwell & Streetly, 2000).

- Patients with SCD often have poor IV access due to repeated
cannulation. The subcutaneous route may be preferable if this is
the case (Newcombe, 2002), as multiple intramuscular injections
can lead to muscle fibrosis. Repeated doses should be given
every 30 min until analgesia is achieved, preferably without
sedation. An effective method of administering subcutaneous or
IV opiates is via a patient-controlled analgesia (PCA) pump.
This allows the patient to self-titrate the drug to their pain (Newcombe, 2002; Butcher, 2004). However, it is unlikely that this
intervention will be instigated in the emergency department.

### Psychological, social and cultural needs

Appropriate professional support can reduce stress and facilitate
coping by offering information, financial help and emotional
support (Atkin & Ahmad, 2000). Despite the many problems
faced by individuals and families, specialist haemoglobinopathy
counsellors provide important support for families, offering co-
ordinated service provision as well as social and emotional
support (Anionwu & Atkin, 2001).

Parents experience a range of emotions when a diagnosis of
sickle cell disorder is given (Bennett, 2005). These include shock,
a sense of failure, disbelief, anger, blame, fear and guilt. The
family is then linked into a structure for on-going care and hospital and community support.

Adults with sickle cell disorders may experience depression
and other psychological problems as a result of the frequency or
intensity of pain. It is possible that depression and other related
problems could increase the incidence and severity of painful
episodes by disrupting coping behaviour (Midence & Elander,
1996). Understanding ethnicity and cultural diversity involves
being aware of different aspects of people's lives such as the
country of origin, religious beliefs, naming systems, language
spoken, dietary habits and practices that can cause medical

problems (Bennett, 2005). Practitioners also need to appreciate the importance of sensitivity in tailoring genetic information and services to the patient's culture, knowledge and language level, recognising that ethnicity, culture, religion and ethical perspectives may influence the patient's ability to use these (Kirk, 2003).

In summary, people with sickle cell disorders are constantly endeavouring to cope with the symptoms of the condition and its impact on their lifestyle. Many people experience sickling crises even when there are no adverse social, psychological or cultural factors. It is important for practitioners to understand that the clinical manifestations of the condition can be associated with social, psychological or cultural factors. Many patients with a sickle cell disorder experience repeated admissions to hospital due to sickling crises. Practitioners should work in collaboration with the patient, keeping them fully informed of interventions and care.

## HYPERTENSIVE CRISIS

An estimated 20% of people in the UK have blood pressure that is elevated to more than 140/90 mmHg, which warrants some form of treatment or monitoring (Elliott, 2002). High blood pressure (hypertension) contributes to the 66,000 deaths from coronary heart disease (CHD) and stroke in people aged under 75 (Department of Health, 1999a), costing the NHS billions of pounds each year (British Heart Foundation, 2002).

The prevalence of high blood pressure is greater in males than in females and rises with age. A Department of Health (1999b) report demonstrated that certain ethnic groups are more prone to hypertension, showing that Black Caribbean and Pakistani women were at least 20% more likely to have high blood pressure than the general female population. Although the incidence of hypertensive crisis is low, affecting fewer than 1% of hypertensive adults, presentation of a patient with severe hypertension to the emergency department demands immediate evaluation, prompt recognition of a hypertensive emergency or urgency, and the prompt initiation of appropriate therapeutic measures to prevent progression of target-organ damage and to avoid a catastrophic event (Bales, 1999).

Hypertensive crisis can occur at any age. It can affect neonates with congenital renal artery hypoplasia, children with acute glomerulonephritis, young pregnant women with eclampsia or elderly people with atherosclerotic renal-artery stenosis. Such individuals are not necessarily accustomed to significant elevations in blood pressure and may present with signs and symptoms of hypertensive emergency at much lower blood pressure levels than patients with chronic hypertension (Webster et al., 1993). Nevertheless, urgent treatment is required.

### Pathogenesis

The factors that lead to the severe and rapid elevation of blood pressure in patients with malignant hypertension are poorly understood. The rapidity of onset suggests a triggering factor (which may be non-specific) superimposed on pre-existing hypertension. The risks for developing malignant hypertension are related to the severity of the underlying hypertension, and therefore the role of mechanical stress on the vessel wall appears to be critical in its pathogenesis (Varon & Marik, 2003). The release of humoral vasoconstrictor substances (particularly the renin–angiotensin axis) is thought to be responsible for the initiation and perpetuation of the hypertensive crisis. Local products produced by the vasculature (e.g. prostaglandins, free radicals) in critically elevated blood pressure may also be involved (Bales, 1999) (Box 4.2).

Crucially, most hypertensive crises are considered to be preventable and are the result of inadequate treatment of mild-to-moderate hypertension or non-adherence to anti-hypertensive therapy. In a few cases, a previously unrecognised form of secondary hypertension, such as renal vascular hypertension or pheochromocytoma, and, rarely, primary hyperaldosteronism, may be responsible and will obviously require early recognition if specific therapy is to be initiated.

---

**Box 4.2 Causes of hypertensive crisis**

Abrupt increase in blood pressure in patients with chronic
   hypertension
Renovascular hypertension
Parenchymal renal disease (chronic)
Scleroderma and other collagen vascular diseases
Use of certain drugs, particularly sympathomimetic agents
   (e.g. cocaine, amphetamines, tricyclic antidepressants;
   especially when combined with monoamino oxidase (MAO)
   inhibitor therapy)
Withdrawal from anti-hypertensive agents (usually centrally
   acting agents)
Pre-eclampsia, eclampsia
Pheochromocytoma
Acute glomerulonephritis
Head injury
Renin-secreting or aldosterone-secreting tumour
Vasculitis
Autonomic hyperactivity in presence of Guillain–Barré or
   other spinal cord syndromes

Sources: Bales (1999) and Calhoun and Oparil (1990).

---

Although hypertension is said to be present when the blood
pressure is 140/90 mmHg or higher (Elliott, 2002), hypertensive
crisis is defined as a critical elevation in blood pressure in which
diastolic pressure exceeds 120 mmHg (Kaplan, 1994). It is characterised by severe accelerated hypertension, accompanied by
evidence of acute or on-going end-organ damage such as coronary ischaemia, disordered cerebral function, a cerebrovascular
event, pulmonary oedema or renal failure (Bales, 1999; Varon &
Marik, 2003).

### Signs and symptoms of hypertensive crisis
Prompt evaluation is needed to identify the clinical status of the
patient, to provide clues to an underlying aetiology of the hypertension, to assess the degree of target organ involvement, and to

select the most appropriate pharmacologic agent and method of administration.

The symptoms and signs of hypertensive crises vary from patient to patient. Symptoms include:

- headache,
- altered level of consciousness,
- focal neurologial signs are seen in patients with hypertensive encephalopathy.

On physical examination, patients may have:

- retinopathy with arteriolar changes, haemorrhages and exudates, as well as papilloedema.

In other patients, the cardiovascular manifestations may predominate:

- angina,
- acute myocardial infarction,
- acute left-ventricular failure.

In some patients, severe injury to the kidneys may lead to acute renal failure with oliguria and/or haematuria.

**Treatment**

Hypertensive emergencies generally require a reduction in blood pressure within a few hours, usually using IV medications given in an intensive care unit (rapid-acting IV agents should not be used outside the intensive care unit because a precipitous and uncontrolled fall in blood pressure may have lethal consequences). All patients with end-organ involvement should have intensive monitoring and have an arterial blood pressure line sited (Vaughan & Delanty, 2000). It should be emphasised that only patients with hypertensive crisis require immediate reduction in markedly elevated blood pressure. In all other patients the elevated blood pressure can be lowered slowly using oral agents.

A variety of different anti-hypertensive agents are available for use in patients with hypertensive crises. The agent(s) of choice will depend on the end organ involved as well as the monitoring environment. There are several anti-hypertensive agents available for this purpose, including:

- esmolol,
- nicardipine,
- labetalol,
- sodium nitroprusside, which is a rapid-acting and potent anti-hypertensive agent; however, it may be associated with significant toxicity and should therefore only be used in select circumstances.

Reductions in diastolic blood pressure by 15–25% or to about 100–110 mmHg is generally recommended. This is best achieved within the first 2 h (Vaughan & Delanty, 2000; Varon & Marik, 2000).

In summary, patients with hypertensive crises may require immediate reduction in elevated blood pressure to prevent and arrest progressive end-organ damage. The best clinical setting in which to achieve this control of blood pressure is in the intensive care unit; therefore, the emergency practitioner holds a key role in patient assessment, history-taking and initial management, which are critical to expedite appropriate transfer and subsequent care.

## DISSECTING AORTIC ANEURYSM

Dissecting aortic aneurysm is a clinical emergency, which carries a high incidence of mortality. Each year there are approximately 3000 people diagnosed with aortic dissection across Europe, and 2000 in the USA (Tsai et al., 2005). It is estimated that aortic aneurysms account for 10,000 deaths each year in the UK (Bick, 2000). Males present more frequently than females (Hagan et al., 2000), having an incidence five to seven times higher (Hatswell, 1994). This is due to protection afforded females by the hormone oestrogen, which inhibits atherosclerosis (Sarrel et al., 1994). An aneurysm can be defined as a local dilatation of a blood vessel. The area of the vessel wall affected becomes progressively weaker as the aneurysm gradually enlarges, and the risk of spontaneous rupture increases. The aorta is one of the large elastic arteries. It originates from the left ventricle of the heart as the thoracic aorta; the abdominal aorta arises at the level of the diaphragm. It then passes inferiorly until it terminates at the bifurcation forming the two common iliac arteries, at around the level of the umbilicus. Several arteries branch off the abdominal aorta, distributing blood to various organs. Thus, it can be seen that the aorta is a crucial structure for normal circulatory function.

### Pathogenesis

Mechanisms which lead to the degeneration and weakening of the medial layers of the aorta can cause higher wall stress and predispose individuals to aneurysm formation and aortic dissection. Results from the International Register of Acute Aortic Dissection (IRAD) (Hagan et al., 2000) suggest that evidence of atherosclerosis may be present in approximately one-third of all patients and highlight the commonest predisposing factor to be hypertension (72%), which may result in ruptured aneurysms in 85% of cases.

Atherosclerosis leads to thickening of the intima, which increases the distance between the endothelial layer and the media; this may compromise nutritional and oxygen supplies, which results in medial thickening and then necrosis. Changes in the elasticity of the medial wall may also lead to vessel stiffness. With the inability to maintain elastic potency, the linings are predisposed to the formation of aneurysms and dissections due to shear wall stress (Neinaber & Eagle, 2003).

Aortic dissection is a tear of the aortic intima that allows the shear forces of blood flow to dissect the intima from the media and, in some instances, penetrate the diseased media with resultant rupture and haemorrhage. Sixty-five per cent of dissections originate within the ascending aorta, 20% within the descending aorta, 10% within the aortic arch and the remainder within the abdominal aorta (Pretre & Von Segesser, 1997).

By the Stanford system, a dissection that involves the ascending aorta is classified as Type A, and one that does not is classified as Type B (European Society of Cardiology Task Force Report, 2001). Dissections are further classified by chronicity as acute (less than 2 weeks) or chronic (greater than 2 weeks); mortality peaks at 2 weeks at approximately 80% and then levels off (Pretre & Von Segesser, 1997).

It has been shown that there is a familial tendency to development of aortic aneurysm (Salo et al., 1999). Lifestyle factors commonly believed to increase the risk of their development are the same as those believed to increase the risk of other forms of arterial disease, such as coronary artery disease and peripheral vascular disease. Smoking is probably the most reported factor associated with an increased risk (Cox, 2007). Other risk factors include high blood cholesterol levels, diabetes mellitus, uncontrolled hypertension and drug abuse (predominantly cocaine abuse).

### Signs and symptoms

The majority of aortic aneurysms are asymptomatic, and present only when they begin to leak or rupture (Bell, 1996). Rupture causes massive haemorrhage into the abdominal cavity, which is usually fatal. Mortality following rupture is more than 90%, with many people dying before they reach hospital (Galland, 1998). In comparison, mortality rates following emergency repair are approximately 50%, and following elective repair are between 5 and 10%; however, survival outcomes are dependent on other factors, for example the age of the patient, the presence of associated renal failure and further complications such as cardiac tamponade (Tsai et al., 2005).

Signs and symptoms of a dissecting aortic aneurysm may be displayed:

- abdominal and/or back pain (Birkitt & Quick, 2002), which may have been present for up to a week, more typical in those with descending-aorta involvement (Hagan et al., 2000);

- chest pain: typically patients describe this as sharp and severe; it is generally more common in patients when the dissection involves the ascending segment of the aorta (Cox, 2007);
- tender, pulsating mass felt on abdominal examination: aneurysms can be difficult to palpate in overweight individuals, and clinical examination has been found to be unreliable (Hatswell, 1994);
- anxiety: may have a sense of 'impending doom';
- syncope: results from the IRAD highlighted that syncope was present in up to 20% of patient with aortic dissection, often indicating the development of serious complications (for example, obstruction to cerebral vessels, cardiac tamponade and neurological impairment) (Hagan et al., 2000).

Many asymptomatic aortic aneurysms are discovered when patients undergo radiological investigations for other conditions, such as ultrasound examination for urological problems.

### Treatment

Essentially the treatment is based upon a rapid early assessment, including history and clinical examination to aid prompt diagnosis, critical, rapid interventions and early transfer to theatre for emergency surgery.

The priorities initially are as follows.

- Assess the patient following the ABCDE approach (Chapter 1). Evaluate MEWS score and alert medics/outreach if necessary (see p. 298).
- If the patient has altered conscious level, their airway is at risk, so summon urgent medical help: this is a rapidly deteriorating life-threatening event.

- Administer high-flow oxygen using a non-rebreathe mask (Figure 1.4). Establish monitoring of oxygen saturation using a pulse oximeter.
- Ensure that the patient has an IV cannula in place.
- Immediate management centres upon reduction of arterial blood pressure. This reduces the force of the left-ventricular ejection pressure, which affects the degree of dissection extension and consequent rupture (Tsai et al., 2005). The lowest tolerable blood pressure should be achieved while maintaining perfusion of other vital organs (Beese-Bjurstrom, 2004), the ideal target range being a systolic pressure of between 100 and 120 mmHg (Tsai et al., 2005).
- Monitor the patient's vital signs closely with frequent re-assessments: deterioration may be rapid; include blood pressure, temperature, pulse and respiratory rate.
- Give appropriate analgesia: morphine sulphate may be used and should be administered in conjunction with an anti-emetic to prevent further aortic trauma due to vomiting (Beese-Bjurstrom, 2004).
- Ensure good communication with the patient, in an attempt to offer re-assurance and thus minimise anxiety and distress.
- Establish continuous ECG monitoring: the patient will be tachycardic. Furthermore, signs of myocardial ischaemia or infarction may be evident, depending on the location and severity of the aortic dissection.
- Request a chest X-ray. This may show widening of the upper mediastinum, a sign that is suggestive of aortic dissection and is present in approximately 60–80% of patients (European Society of Cardiology Task Force Report, 2001).
- Computerised tomography scan (CT scan) may be advocated depending on the patient's stability and condition; this has a sensitivity of greater than 90% and a specificity of 85%.
- Patients with Stanford Type A (ascending) dissection are deemed surgical emergencies, and treatment will help

prevent aortic rupture and the development of pericardial effusion which may lead to cardiac tamponade. Medical management alone is associated with increased mortality (European Society of Cardiology Task Force Report, 2001).

- Prepare for immediate transfer to theatre for immediate surgical repair; following consent by the surgical team present. Transthoracic echocardiography (TTE) and transoesophageal echocardiography (TOE) can be used in the emergency- or operating-department settings.

In summary, a dissecting aortic aneurysm is a clinical emergency which can progress to life-threatening aortic rupture which is particularly distressing and frightening for the patient and carer. A good understanding of the assessment and care is essential to ensure appropriate management of the patient.

## REFERENCES

Anderson, FA & Spencer, FA (2003) Risk factors for venous thromboembolism. *Circulation* **107**(23), suppl 1, 19–16

Anionwu, E & Atkin, K (2001) *The Politics of Sickle Cell and Thalassaemia*. Open University Press, Maidenhead

Atkin, K & Ahmad, W (2000) Family care-giving and chronic illness: how parents cope with a child with sickle cell disorder or thalassaemia. *Health and Social Care in the Community* **8**(1), 57

Bales, A (1999) Hypertensive crisis: How to tell if it's an emergency or an urgency. *Postgraduate Medicine* **105**(5), 39–45

Beese-Bjurstrom, B (2004) Aortic aneurysms and dissections. *Nursing* **34**(2), 36–41

Bell, P (1996) Leaking abdominal aortic aneurysms. *Care of the Critically Ill* **12**(2), 59–63

Bennett, L (2005) Understanding sickle cell disorders. *Nursing Standard* **19**(32), 52–61

Bick, C (2000) Abdominal aortic aneurysm repair. *Nursing Standard* **15**(3), 47–52

Birkitt, HG & Quick, CRG (2002) *Essential Surgery*, 3rd edn. Churchill Livingstone, London

British Heart Foundation (2002) *True Cost of Heart Disease*. www.heartstats.org/uploads/documents%5CHeartFailure2002.pdf (accessed 6 July 2007)

British National Formulary (2005) *British National Formulary no. 49*. British Medical Association and Royal Pharmaceutical Society of Great Britain, London

British Thoracic Society Standards of Care Committee Pulmonary Embolism Guideline Development Group (2003) British Thoracic Society guidelines for the management of suspected acute pulmonary embolism. *Thorax* **58**(6), 470–83

Brooker, C (1998) *Human Structure and Function, Nursing Application and clinical Practice*, 2nd edn. Mosby, London

Butcher, D (2004) Pharmacological techniques in managing acute pain in emergency departments. *Emergency Nurse* **12**(1), 26–36

Calhoun, DA & Oparil, S (1990) Treatment of hypertensive crisis. *New England Journal of Medicine* **323**(17), 1177–83

Claster, S & Vichinsky, EP (2003) Managing sickle cell disease. *British Medical Journal* **327**(7424), 1151–5

Cox, H (2007) Assessing and managing the patient with chest pain due to an aortic dissection. In Albarran, J & Tagney, J (eds), *Chest Pain.* Blackwell Publishing, Oxford

Department of Health (1999a) *Saving Lives: Our Healthier Nation*. Department of Health, London

Department of Health (1999b) *The Health Survey for England: the Health of Minority Ethnic Groups '99*. Department of Health, London

Eboh, W (1996) Sickle cell disease. *Practice Nursing* **7**(1), 25–7

Elliott, H (2002) Epidemiology, aetiology and prognosis of hypertension. *Medicine Student Edition* **30**(7), 127–130

Enders, JM, Burke, JM & Dobesh, PP (2002) Prevention of venous thromboembolism in acute medical illness. *Pharmacotherapy* **22**(12), 1564–78

European Society of Cardiology Task Force Report (2001) Diagnosis and management of aortic dissection. *European Heart Journal* **22**, 897–903

Galland, RB (1998) Problems associated with aortic surgery. *Care of the Critically Ill* **14**(2), 51–5

Gerotziafas, GT & Samama, MM (2004) Prophylaxis of venous thromboembolism in medical patients. *Current Opinion in Pulmonary Medicine* **10**(5), 356–65

Gorman, WP, Davis, KR & Donnelly, R (2000) ABC of arterial and venous disease. Swollen lower limb-1: general assessment and deep vein thrombosis. *British Medical Journal* **3320**(7247), 1453–6

Hagan PG, Nienaber CA, Isselbacher EM, Bruckman D, Karavite DJ, Russman PL, et al. (2000) The International Register of Acute Aortic Dissection (IRAD). New insights into an old disease. *Journal of the American Medical Association* **283**(7), 897–903

Hatswell, E (1994) Abdominal aortic surgery. Part 1: An overview and discussion of immediate peri-operative complications. *Heart and Lung* **23**(3), 228–39

Hinchliff, SM (1996) *Physiology for Nursing Practice*, 2nd edn. Baillière Tindall, London

House of Commons Health Committee (2005) *The Prevention of Venous Thromboembolism in Hospitalised Patients.* www.publications.parliament.uk/pa/cm200405/cmselect/cmhealth/99/99.pdf (accessed 6 July 2007)

Kakkar, VV & De Lorenzo, F (1998) Prevention of venous thromboembolism in general surgery. *Baillieres Clinical Haematolology* **11**, 605–19

Kaplan, NM (1994) Management of hypertensive emergencies. *Lancet* **344**(8933), 1335–8

Kirk, M (2003) *Fit For Practice in the Genetics Era: a Competence based Education Framework for Nurses, Midwives and Health Visitors.* Genomics Policy Unit, University of Glamorgan, and the Medical Genetics Service for Wales, University Hospital of Wales

Kumar, P & Clark, M (2002) *Clinical Medicine*, 5th edn. WB Saunders and Co, London

Levine, M, Gent, M, Hirsh, J, Leclerc, J & Anderson, D (1996) Treatment of venous thrombosis with intravenous unfractionated heparin, administered in hospital as compared with subcutaneous LMWH administered at home. *New England Journal of Medicine* **334**(11), 677–81

Lewis, SM & Collier, IC (1992) *Medical-Surgical Nursing Assessment and Management of Clinical Problems*, 3rd edn. Mosby, St Louis, MO

Marieb, HN (1998) *Human Anatomy and Physiology*, 4th edn. Benjamin Cummings, Menlo Park, CA

Maxwell, K & Streetly, A (2000) *Living with Sickle Pain*. Guy's, King's and St Thomas' School of Medicine, London

McColl, MD, Ramsay, JE, Tait, RC, Walker, ID, McCall, F & Conkie, JA (1997) Risk factors for pregnancy associated venous thromboembolism. *Thrombosis and Haemostasis* **78**, 1183–8

McKenzie, S (1996) *Textbook of Haematology*, 2nd edn. Williams and Wilkins, Baltimore, MD

Mehta, A & Hoffbrand, V (2000) *Haematology at a Glance*. Blackwell Science, Oxford

Midence, K & Elander, J (1996) Adjustment and coping in adults with sickle cell disease: an assessment of research evidence. *British Journal of Health Psychology* **1**, 95–111

Modell, B (2005) World distribution of haemoglobin gene variants. *Scandinavian Journal of Clinical and Laboratory Investigations* **67**(1), 39–70

Murray, N & May, A (1988) Painful crises in sickle cell disease – patients' perspectives. *British Medical Journal* **297**, 452–4

Newcombe, P (2002) Pathophysiology of sickle cell disease crisis. *Emergency Nurse* **9**(9), 19–22

Neinaber, C & Eagle, K (2003) Aortic dissection: new frontiers in diagnosis and management. Part 1. From etiology to diagnostic strategies. *Circulation* **108**, 628–35

Pretre, R & Von Segesser, LK (1997) Aortic dissection. *Lancet* **349**(9063), 1461–4

Robinson, GV (2006) Pulmonary embolism in hospital practice. *British Medical Journal* **332**(21), 156–60

Salo, JA, Soisalon-Soininen, S & Mattila, PS (1999) Familial occurrences of abdominal aortic aneurysm. *Annals of Internal Medicine* **130**(8), 637–42

Sarrel, P, Lufkin, EG, Oursler, MJ & Keefe, D (1994) Oestrogen actions in arteries, bone and brain. *Science and Medicine* **1**(3), 44–53

Streetly, A (2004) *Information for Community Practitioners: the NHS Sickle Cell and Thalassaemia Screening Programme.* www.kclphs. org.uk/haemscreening/Documents/CommPracInfo.pdf (accessed 4 April 2005)

Tortora, G & Anagnostakos, P (2000) *Principles of Anatomy and Physiology*, 9th edn. Harper & Rowe, New York

Tovey, C & Wyatt, S (2003) Diagnosis, investigation, and management of deep vein thrombosis. *British Medical Journal* **326**(7400), 1180–4

Tsai, T, Neinaber, C & Kin, K (2005) Acute aortic syndromes. *Circulation* **112**(24), 3802–13

Turpie, AG, Chin, BS & Lip, GY (2002) Venous thromboembolism: pathophysiology, clinical features, and prevention. *British Medical Journal* **325**(7369), 887–90

United Kingdom Venous Thromboembolism Registry (VERITY) (2004) Venous thromboembolism. Registry Second Annual Report. *Hospital Medicine* **65**(5), 260–1

Urbano, FL (2001) Homans' sign in the diagnosis of deep venous thrombosis. *Hospital Physician* **98**(5), 22–4

Varon, J & Marik, PE (2000) The diagnosis and management of hypertensive crises. *Chest* **118**, 214–27

Varon, J & Marik, PE (2003) Clinical review: the management of hypertensive crises. *Critical Care* **7**(5), 374–84

Vaughan, CJ & Delanty, N (2000) Hypertensive emergencies. *Lancet* **356**(9239), 411–17

Wallis, M & Autar, R (2001) Deep vein thrombosis: clinical nursing management. *Nursing Standard* **15**(18), 47–54

Webster, J, Petrie, JC & Jeffers, TA (1993) Accelerated hypertension: patterns of mortality and clinical factors affecting outcome in treated patients. *Quarterly Journal of Medicine* **86**(8), 485–93

Welch, E (2006) The assessment and management of venous thromboembolism. *Nursing Standard* **20**(28), 58–64

# 5 Shock

Beverley Ewens

## INTRODUCTION

Shock is an altered physiological state that can affect every functioning cell in the body. It is a complex syndrome which reflects decreased perfusion to tissues resulting in cellular dysfunction and ultimately organ failure (Elliott et al., 2007). The aim of this chapter is to allow the reader to understand the different manifestations of shock and its management.

## LEARNING OUTCOMES

At the end of the chapter the reader will be able to:

❏ differentiate between distributive, obstructive, cardiogenic and hypovolaemic shock,
❏ discuss the different management plans for each,
❏ explain the use and complications of vasopressor/inotrope drug therapy.

## DISTRIBUTIVE SHOCK

Distributive shock results from maldistribution of blood volume and decreased oxygen uptake at the cellular level (Mower-Wade et al., 2001). There are three categories of distributive shock:

• septic,
• anaphylactic,
• neurogenic.

These types of shock are caused by a reduction in systemic vascular resistance secondary to massive vasodilation. Whether caused by systemic infection, anaphylaxis or spinal nerve damage the patient will feel peripherally warm because of the vasodilation and the inability to compensate for this (Bench, 2004).

## Sepsis

Sepsis is a common and frequently fatal condition (DeMarco & MacArthur, 2006) affecting 18 million people worldwide every year (Slade et al., 2003), and its incidence is increasing (Russell, 2006). Morbidity and mortality rates remain unacceptably high (Dellinger et al., 2004; Poeze et al., 2004; Vincent & Abraham, 2006; Sevransky et al., 2007), reported to be 30–40% (DeMarco & MacArthur, 2006), and the condition accounts for 10% of all admissions to the intensive care unit (ICU) (Annane et al., 2005).

Sepsis can be a rapidly fatal condition and it is believed that the management of the patient in an initial '6-hour window' impacts significantly upon mortality and morbidity, during which time specific goal-directed therapy is advocated (Rivers et al., 2001; Dellinger et al., 2004; Rhodes & Bennett, 2004; King, 2007). It is therefore essential that nurses monitor patients appropriately, recognise the emerging signs of shock and communicate findings accordingly.

### Definitions

In 1992 the American College of Chest Physicians (ACCP) and the Society of Critical Care Medicine (SCCM) defined a practical framework to define the systemic inflammatory response to syndrome (SIRS) (Levy et al., 2003). SIRS is an acronym for the complex findings that result from a systemic activation of the immune response (Levy et al., 2003) (Table 5.1). SIRS can be self-limiting or can progress to severe sepsis or septic shock (Rivers et al., 2001).

Guidelines on the relevance of SIRS in clinical diagnosis of sepsis are given below.

Sepsis:

- two or more SIRS criteria,
- confirmed or suspected infection.

**Table 5.1** The systemic inflammatory response to infection (SIRS) criteria

| Core temperature >38.3 or <36°C | |
|---|---|
| Heart rate | >90 beats/min |
| Respiratory rate | >20 breaths/min or $PaCO_2$ <4.3 kPa (32 mmHg) |
| White blood count | <4000 or >12,000 $\mu l^{-1}$ |

Source: Bone et al. (1992).

Supporting criteria for diagnosis are: hyperglycaemia, altered mental status, raised lactate and reduced capillary refill time.

Severe sepsis:

- two or more SIRS criteria,
- organ dysfunction (Levy et al., 2003) (Table 5.2),
- hypotension or poor perfusion (before fluid challenge).

Septic shock:

- severe sepsis with hypotension (systolic blood pressure <90 mmHg) despite adequate fluid resuscitation (Levy et al., 2003), i.e., 20–40 mls/kg,
- unexplained metabolic acidosis (blood pH <7.35; $HCO^{3-}$ <20 mmol/l; base excess >2.5 mmol/l),
- decreased capillary-refill time or mottled/cool extremities (Levy et al., 2003).

**Sepsis and organ dysfunction**

*Pathogenesis*

The pathogenesis of sepsis involves several factors that interact in a long chain of events from pathogen recognition to the overwhelming of the host response (Annane et al., 2005) and is remarkably complex (Parrillo, 2005). The early stages of sepsis are characterised by an excess of inflammatory mediators but as the condition progresses immunosuppression becomes the dominating feature (Das, 2006). The immune system response is dependent on many factors, including extremes of age, virulence of organisms, health status, nutritional status and immune-receptor response (Kleinpell et al., 2006). Inflammation is a normal physio-

**Table 5.2** Sepsis and organ dysfunction

| System | Physiological manifestation | May progress to |
| --- | --- | --- |
| Cardiovascular system | SBP <90 mmHg<br>Mean arterial pressure (MAP)<br>  <60 mmHg or SBP <40 mmHg<br>  less than patient's normal value<br>  in the absence of other causes<br>Poor perfusion and/or mottled skin<br>Raised blood lactate level<br>  (>2 mmol/l) | Low cardiac output syndrome<br>Ischaemic bowel<br>Acute tubular necrosis (ATN)<br>Limb/digit necrosis<br>Severe metabolic acidosis<br>MODS |
| Central nervous system | Altered mental state; confusion, psychosis | |
| Respiratory system | Tachypnoea<br>Hypoxaemia: $SpO_2$ <93% or $PaO_2$<br>  <9 kPa (67 mmHg) | Acute respiratory distress syndrome (ARDS)<br>Acute lung injury (ALI) |
| Endocrine system | Hyperglycaemia in the absence of diabetes | |
| Renal system | Oliguria and/or raised urea and creatinine | Acute renal failure |
| Coagulation | INR >1.5, APTT >60 s or platelets <100 µl<br>Platelet count <100 µl<br>White blood count <4000 or >12,000 $\mu l^{-1}$ | Disseminated intravascular coagulation (DIC)<br>Stroke |
| Gastrointestinal tract | Gastric stasis, i.e. ileus<br>Abnormal liver function tests<br>Jaundice<br>Increased D-dimer levels | Acute liver failure |

Adapted from Robson and Newell (2005), Smith (2005) and King (2007).
APTT, activated partial thromboplastin time; INR, international normalised ratio; MODS, multiple organ dysfunction syndrome; SBP, systolic blood pressure.

logical response to bacteria and viruses and consists of three localised stages: vasodilation and increased blood-vessel permeability, emigration of phagocytes and tissue repair (Robson & Newell, 2005). In sepsis the normal inflammatory immune response is accelerated and the normal anti-inflammatory systems in the body cease to function (King, 2007). How the host responses function and the characteristics of the infecting organism influence the outcome of sepsis (Russell, 2006). Microorganisms proliferate at the central point of infection and the organism or toxin enters the body (Parrillo, 2005). Inflammatory mediators are released from plasma proteins (the coagulation, fibrinolytic and complement systems) or from cells (endothelial, monocyte macrophages and neutrophils) (Parrillo, 2005). These mediators have a profound affect on the vasculature and multi-organ systems.

This results in a widening of the vasculature and fluid loss out of the circulation, resulting in a reduction in blood pressure. The coagulation system becomes activated and microthrombi form in the blood vessels (Robson & Newell, 2005). These microthrombi impede blood flow to tissues and in combination with reduced organ perfusion lead to multiple organ dysfunction syndrome (MODS) (Robson & Newell, 2005). Most patients who die from septic shock do so because of MODS (Ahrens, 2006).

*Causes*

The organisms that can cause sepsis are extensive and include:

- bacteria, Gram-negative and Gram-positive (85% of all cases),
- viruses,
- fungi (mortality 40%),
- parasites.

Common causes of sepsis:

- respiratory tract: pneumonia, empyema;
- cardiovascular: endocarditis;
- intra-abdominal: pancreatitis, ischaemic gut, peritonitis;
- neurological: meningitis, encephalitis, cerebral abscess;
- skin: necrotising fasciitis, insect bites, wound infection, pressure sores;
- urinary tract: pyelonephritis;
- skeleton: osteomyelitis;
- reproductive: missed abortion, pelvic inflammatory disease, toxic shock syndrome;
- line sepsis: central venous catheters, chest drains.

(Sources: Robson & Newell, 2005; Smith, 2005)

*Clinical features of sepsis*

Hyperthermia or hypothermia, tachycardia, wide pulse pressure, tachypnoea and unexplained changes in mental health status are all early systemic signs of infection and septic shock (Jui, 2004). The three stages of shock have been described as:

- compensated: body mechanisms are triggered to maintain adequate blood pressure for perfusion;
- progressive: compensatory mechanisms begin to fail and reduced organ perfusion become apparent;
- irreversible: refractory shock which does not respond to treatment.

(Source: Bench, 2004)

*Investigations*

Investigations that should be undertaken include:

- routine bloods: urea, electrolytes and creatinine, full blood count, glucose;
- liver function tests, clotting screen;
- cultures of blood, urine, sputum, wound;
- C-reactive protein (CRP), D-dimer;
- arterial blood gas, including lactate;
- radiological investigations, such as chest X-ray, abdominal X-ray, CT scan and MRI scan.

(Sources: Robson & Newell, 2005; Smith, 2005)

*Diagnosis*

Diagnosis is based upon clinical presentation and course of illness. Treatment should be commenced prior to the identification of any organism to improve outcomes from sepsis.

*Treatment of sepsis*

The treatment of sepsis must be based on best evidence and early goal-directed therapy is recognised as the cornerstone of early management because early recognition and early aggressive treatment using evidence-based guidelines can save lives (Robson

& Newell, 2005; Russell, 2006). It is recommended that patients with sepsis are managed in a higher-care facility such as a high-dependency unit (HDU) or an intensive care unit (ICU), where both invasive and non-invasive monitoring can be utilised (Maier, 2005; Robson & Newell, 2005), enabling detailed continuous assessment of the patient's physiological state (Maier, 2005).

- Assess the patient using the ABCDE approach as (Chapter 1). Evaluate MEWS score, alert medical staff/outreach team if necessary (see p. 298).
- Early high-flow oxygen therapy via a non-rebreathe mask should be commenced (Bench, 2004).
- Insert an arterial pressure monitoring line for continuous arterial pressure monitoring. Insert a urinary catheter to assess hourly urine output (Maier, 2005).
- Insert a central venous catheter (CVC) to facilitate fluid resuscitation and central venous pressure (CVP) reading.
- Takes cultures of blood, urine, sputum, etc. prior to commencing antibiotic treatment.
- Treat or remove the source of infection (e.g. culture appropriate sites, remove indwelling devices, drain collections, surgery for ischaemic bowel) (Bench, 2004; Robson & Newell, 2005; Powers & Jacobi, 2006).
- Commence appropriate antibiotics, based on clinical judgment.
- Early goal-directed therapy has been demonstrated to improve survival by 16% (Rivers et al., 2001; Dellinger et al., 2004) and refers to the specific resuscitation of severely septic patients or in septic shock immediately at presentation to hospital (Rivers et al., 2001; Rhodes & Bennett, 2004). Fluids and vasopressors/inotropic drugs are administered to maintain the following physiological parameters: CVP 8–12 mmHg, mean arterial pressure >65 and <90 mmHg, haematocrit >30%, central venous oxygen saturation ($SvO_2$) ≥70%.
- Commence invasive ventilation for those patients who cannot be optimised by the preceding treatments (Rivers et al., 2001).

- Consider administration of recombinant human activated protein C in septic shock, sepsis-induced acute respiratory distress syndrome (ARDS) and sepsis-induced MODS (Fourrier, 2004).
- Maintain blood glucose levels at <8.3 mmol/l (Parrillo, 2005).
- Start renal replacement therapy where indicated.
- Administer corticosteroids if the patient has proven adrenal insufficiency.

*Complications of sepsis*

- ARDS
- Acute renal failure
- Hepatic failure
- MODS

*Pharmacologic support of shock*

The role of inotropes (which increase the force of cardiac contraction) and vasopressors (which cause vasoconstriction) is often vital in the management of advanced shock of any aetiology. All of these drugs act on the sympathetic nervous system but the effect varies depending on which sympathetic receptor the drug has the greatest affinity for (Gilmore & Nanyanzi, 1999) (Table 5.3). All patients receiving vasopressor/inotrope therapy require continuous ECG monitoring and continuous pulse oximetry. Invasive arterial pressure monitoring is preferable.

### Noradrenaline (norepinephrine)

Noradrenaline is the most commonly used vasopressor in sepsis as it has powerful vasoconstrictor properties and is less likely to cause tachycardia than adrenaline (Gilmore & Nanyanzi, 1999). Because of its vasoconstrictor effects noradrenaline increases afterload and is therefore not used in cardiogenic shock. Blood supply to peripheries and kidneys may be impaired and in severe cases this can lead to ischaemia and necrosis of digits and/or limbs. Noradrenaline is administered via a central venous catheter (CVC) by continual infusion because of its short half-life.

**Table 5.3** Inotropes/vasopressors and receptor sites

|  | Alpha₁ (peripheral arteriolar vasoconstriction) | Alpha₂ | Beta₁ (increased heart rate and force of contraction) | Beta₂ (bronchial smooth muscle dilation, skeletal muscle vasodilation) | Dopamine (increased renal blood flow) |
|---|---|---|---|---|---|
| Dobutamine | + | + | ++++ | ++ | 0 |
| Dopamine | ++/+++ | ? | ++++ | ++ | ++++ |
| Adrenaline | ++++ | ++++ | ++++ | +++ | 0 |
| Noradrenaline | +++ | +++ | +++ | +/++ | 0 |

Source: Gilmore and Nanyanzi (1999).

### Adrenaline (epinephrine)

Adrenaline prepares the body for 'fight and flight' by increasing cardiac contractility and heart rate, thereby increasing cardiac output (Gilmore & Nanyazi, 1999). Side effects include hypertension, tachycardia and cardiac arrhythmias. At higher doses vasoconstriction occurs, leading to cool peripheries.

### Dobutamine

Dobutamine increases cardiac output by its inotropic effect but it also reduces afterload. This makes dobutamine a useful drug in cardiogenic shock where afterload is increased. Dobutamine can be administered peripherally.

### Dopamine

Dopamine is the natural precursor of noradrenaline and adrenaline in the body. It is less frequently used in clinical practice now. Low-dose dopamine (1–2 µg/kg per min) does not prevent renal damage as was once thought. Higher doses of dopamine (>2 µg/kg per min) increase cardiac contractility. Side effects include tachycardia.

**Anaphylaxis**

Anaphylaxis is a potentially life-threatening condition that nurses may encounter while practising in any sphere of nursing (Ferns & Chojnacka, 2003). Although anaphylaxis is on the increase confusion about treatment, recognition and investigations and follow up persists, despite previous guidelines (Resuscitation Council UK, 2008).

The prevalence of anaphylaxis is unclear, which is due primarily to under-reporting and poor definition (Finney & Rushton, 2007), although estimates of mortality are 10–20 people per year in England (Bryant, 2007). Anaphylaxis is a rapidly progressing sequelae of events that is potentially fatal (Evans & Tippins, 2005). Nursing staff require an in-depth knowledge of the presentation and management of anaphylaxis to maximise the chance of recovery (Ferns & Chojnacka, 2003).

*Pathogensis*

Anaphylaxis is the end result of an allergic reaction following re-exposure to a substance or antigen (Crusher, 2004) which leads to an excessive and inappropriate immune response (Finney & Rushton, 2007), although no universally accepted definition exists (Resuscitation Council UK, 2008). The immune system is activated when proteins (immunoglobulins or antibodies) react with foreign proteins (antigens) (Bryant, 2007). During initial contact with the antigen plasma cells make specific immunoglobulin E (IgE) antibodies that attach to mast cells and basophils, which then lie dormant (Crusher, 2004). When the body re-encounters the antigen, IgE recognises it and an allergic reaction takes place as mediators are released from the mast cells and basophils (Ferns & Chojnacka, 2003). These chemical mediators include histamine, tryptase and leukotrines, which lead to the contraction of smooth muscle, increase in vascular permeability and reduction in systemic vascular resistance due to intravascular fluid loss into the extravascular space.

*Causes*

The most common causes of anaphylaxis are:

- therapeutic drugs (62%),
- food (15%),
- insect venom (11%).

(Source: Sheikh & Alves, 2001)

See also Table 5.4.

### Clinical features
Anaphylaxis can manifest itself in many ways (Crusher, 2004). Clinical features include:

- hay fever symptoms, due to histamine release;
- urticaria, pruritis, erythema;
- a metallic taste in the mouth;
- altered level of consciousness;
- angio-oedema, caused by dilation and increased permeability of the capillaries, may lead to upper-airway obstruction;

**Table 5.4** Causes of anaphylaxis

| Cause | Examples |
|---|---|
| Drugs | Penicillin and cephalosporins |
| | Aspirin and non-steroidal anti-inflammatory drugs |
| | Anaesthetic agents |
| | Opiates |
| | Progesterone |
| | Insulin |
| | Streptokinase |
| | Vaccinations |
| Blood products | |
| Latex | |
| Food | Nuts |
| | Fish |
| | Shellfish |
| | Eggs |
| | Dairy products |
| Insect stings and bites | Wasps and hornets |
| | Honey and bumble bees |
| Intravenous contrast medium (anaphylactoid reaction, identical to anaphylaxis) | |
| Plasma expanders | |

Sources: Ferns and Chojnacka (2003), Crusher (2004) and Jevon (2006).

- bronchospasm, stridor, dyspnoea;
- tachycardia, arrhythmias and hypotension, due to loss of intravascular volume;
- anxiety, restlessness, feeling of 'impending doom';
- abdominal pain, nausea and vomiting.

(Sources; Ferns & Chojnacka, 2003; Bryant, 2007)

*Diagnosis*

In each case a full history and examination must be undertaken as soon as possible. Special attention should be given to the condition of the skin, heart rate, blood pressure, upper airways and auscultation of the chest (Resuscitation Council UK, 2008). Anaphylaxis can often be confused with panic attacks or vasovagal episodes. Although an anxiety-related erythematous rash may be present, other signs of anaphylaxis will be absent (Jevon, 2006) (Table 5.5). Expertise in management and early treatment is paramount (Ferns & Chojnacka, 2003).

Detailed assessment using the ABCDE method is recommended, as follows.

- Airway: ensure that the airway is patent, assess for any obstructions, such as the tongue or dentures. Listen for stridor or wheeze and for the presence of angio-oedema. Apply high-flow oxygen via a non-rebreathe mask. Commence continuous pulse oximetry.

**Table 5.5** Conditions with a similar presentation to anaphylaxis

| Condition | Vasovagal attack | Anxiety attack | Asthma attack |
|---|---|---|---|
| Similarities to anaphylaxis | Hypotension, anxiety and respiratory distress | Tachycardia, palpitations and dyspnoea | Respiratory distress and tachycardia |
| Differences to anaphylaxis | Bradycardia likely and pale in colour | Absence of urticaria or hypotension | Absence of facial flushing or urticaria |

Source: Finney and Rushton (2007).

147

- Breathing: assess the depth and rate of respirations by auscultation and visual inspection.
- Circulation: assess the capillary refill time; a time of greater than 2 seconds will indicate poor peripheral perfusion. Feel for the rate and quality of the pulse, and monitor ECG and blood pressure. Hypotension indicates the necessity for urgent treatment as cardiac output is compromised.
- Disability: utilise the AVPU scale (described in Chapter 6) as a quick assessment of the patient's level of consciousness.
- Exposure: expose the patient and observe the skin for colour, pallor, urticaric rash and/or swelling.

### *Treatment*

Evidence-based treatment guidelines for anaphylaxis are outlined in Figure 5.1.

- Assess the patient following the ABCDE approach described in chapter 1.
- Evaluate MEWS score and contact medical staff/outreach team where necessary (see p. 298).
- Adrenaline: this is the most important treatment for anaphylaxis and is indicated for bronchospasm, laryngeal oedema, hypotension, urticaria and angio-oedema. Intramuscular adrenaline (500 mcg IM) is sufficient in most cases, repeated at 5-min intervals until a response is seen. Adrenaline reverses vasodilation, reduces oedema, dilates the bronchioles, inhibits further mediator response and has an inotropic effect on the myocardium.
- Antihistamine: chlorpheniramine or phenergan should be used routinely as they help counter histamine-mediated vasodilation.
- Intravenous fluids: indicated for hypotension. These will replace intravascular fluid lost into the extravascular space.
- Corticosteroids: these may help in the emergency treatment of an acute attack and play a role in preventing or shortening protracted reactions. They are particularly useful in patients with asthma.

(Sources: Crusher, 2004; Resuscitation Council UK, 2008)

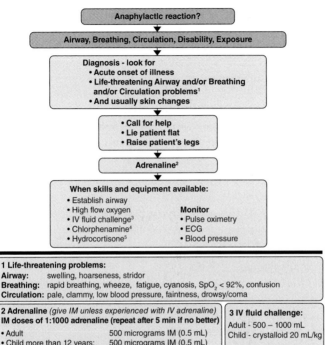

| | Anaphylactic reaction? |
|---|---|

**Airway, Breathing, Circulation, Disability, Exposure**

**Diagnosis - look for**
- **Acute onset of illness**
- **Life-threatening Airway and/or Breathing and/or Circulation problems[1]**
- **And usually skin changes**

- **Call for help**
- **Lie patient flat**
- **Raise patient's legs**

**Adrenaline[2]**

**When skills and equipment available:**
- Establish airway
- High flow oxygen
- IV fluid challenge[3]
- Chlorphenamine[4]
- Hydrocortisone[5]

**Monitor**
- Pulse oximetry
- ECG
- Blood pressure

**1 Life-threatening problems:**
**Airway:** swelling, hoarseness, stridor
**Breathing:** rapid breathing, wheeze, fatigue, cyanosis, $SpO_2$ < 92%, confusion
**Circulation:** pale, clammy, low blood pressure, faintness, drowsy/coma

**2 Adrenaline** *(give IM unless experienced with IV adrenaline)*
**IM doses of 1:1000 adrenaline (repeat after 5 min if no better)**

| | |
|---|---|
| • Adult | 500 micrograms IM (0.5 mL) |
| • Child more than 12 years: | 500 micrograms IM (0.5 mL) |
| • Child 6 – 12 years: | 300 micrograms IM (0.3 mL) |
| • Child less than 6 years: | 150 micrograms IM (0.15 mL) |

Adrenaline IV to be given **only by experienced specialists**
Titrate: Adults 50 micrograms; Children 1 microgram/kg

**3 IV fluid challenge:**
Adult - 500 – 1000 mL
Child - crystalloid 20 mL/kg

Stop IV colloid
if this might be the cause
of anaphylaxis

| | 4 Chlorphenamine | 5 Hydrocortisone |
|---|---|---|
| | (IM or slow IV) | (IM or slow IV) |
| Adult or child more than 12 years | 10 mg | 200 mg |
| Child 6 – 12 years | 5 mg | 100 mg |
| Child 6 months to 6 years | 2.5 mg | 50 mg |
| Child less than 6 months | 250 micrograms/kg | 25 mg |

**Figure 5.1** Emergency treatment of anaphylactic reactions. Guidelines for healthcare providers. Resuscitation Council UK (2008).
ALS, advanced life support; CPR, cardiopulmonary resuscitation; IM, intramuscular; IV, intravenous.

**Neurogenic shock**

Neurogenic shock is a form of distributive shock caused by loss of vasomotor (sympathetic) tone, due to inhibition of neural output (Elliott et al., 2007). Neurogenic shock is less common than other forms of distributive shock but should be considered if patients present with spinal injury or have received spinal anaesthesia (Bench, 2004). Neurogenic shock must not be confused with spinal shock, when a temporary loss of spinal reflex activity occurs below a total or near-total spinal cord injury (Eurle & Scalea, 2004).

*Causes*

The primary cause of neurogenic shock is spinal injury above thoracic vertebra 6 (T6), secondary to the disruption of sympathetic outflow from T1 to lumbar vertebra 2 (L2). It may also be secondary to disruption of the thoracic sympathetic outflow tract when there is partial or complete injury above it (Elliott et al., 2007).

*Pathophysiology*

Block of the sympathetic nervous system allows the parasympathetic system to dominate, resulting in reduced vasomotor tone, pooling of blood in dilated capacitance vessels, reduced venous return and reduced cardiac output.

*Clinical features*

Hypotension that is characteristic of neurogenic shock usually begins within 5 min of injury to the spinal cord (Elliott et al., 2007):

- hypotension, due to a reduction in systemic vascular resistance and venous return;
- the patient may have warm dry skin;
- bradycardia, due to dominance of the parasympathetic system (vagus nerve);
- flaccid paralysis, including bowel and bladder;
- hypothermia, due to vasodilation.

*Treatment*

If the patient has sustained a spinal injury, early recognition and immobilization of the spine will help prevent further worsening of the condition (Eurle & Scalea, 2004).

- Assess the patient following the ABCDE approach described in chapter 1.
- Evaluate MEWS score and contact medical staff/outreach team where necessary (see p. 298).
- Position the patient supine with spinal immobilisation.
- Administer high-flow oxygen.
- Ensure continuous monitoring of vital signs.
- Insert a urinary catheter.
- Allow for rapid infusion of fluids, preferably via a CVC.
- Administer chronotropic agents, for example atropine for bradycardia or temporary pacing for complete heart block.
- Initiate vasopressor (noradrenaline) therapy to maintain adequate mean arterial pressure.

*Complications*

Complications of neurogenic shock include:

- deep-vein thrombosis (DVT),
- MODS.

## HYPOVOLAEMIC SHOCK

Hypovolaemia is the most common form of shock. When the body loses circulating volume, venous return to the heart decreases and compensatory mechanisms involving catecholamine release and increases in sympathetic drive result in the initial changes of tachycardia and cool skin but have little effect on cardiac and cerebral vessels (Mower-Wade et al., 2001). If left untreated hypovolaemic shock can lead to inadequate tissue perfusion, cellular damage and ultimately MODS (Hughes, 2004). Sometimes the cause of loss of circulating volume is obvious, as in haemorrhage, but at other times it can be less so, as in cases of loss of fluid from the gut due to paralytic ileus (Collins, 2000). It is important to note that in healthy individuals 30% of circulating volume can be lost before compensatory mechanisms can no longer counterbalance such losses and physiological disturbance becomes apparent (Table 5.6).

**Table 5.6** Four classifications of hypovolaemic shock

| Blood loss | Observations |
|---|---|
| Class 1 (>15% blood volume, 750 ml) | Usually few signs; this is a compensatory stage to attempt to overcome the shock: HR <100 beats/min, normal BP, respiratory rate 14–20 breaths/min, urinary output normal |
| Class 2 (15–30% blood volume, 750–1500 ml) | HR >100 beats/min (pulse will be thready), normal BP, respiratory rate 20–30 breaths/min, reduced urine output of 20–30 ml/h, cool skin |
| Class 3 (30–40% blood volume, 1500–2000 ml) | Dramatic deterioration in vital signs: HR >120 beats/min, BP decreased, respiratory rate 30–40 breaths/min, urinary output 5–15 ml/h, anxiety and confusion |
| Class 4 (>40% blood volume, >2000 ml) | Immediate threat to patient's life: HR >140 beats/min, BP decreased, respiratory rate >40 breaths/min, urinary output <5 ml/h, confusion and lethargy |

Sources: American College of Surgeons (1993), cited in Collins (2000) and Mower-Wade et al. (2001).
BP, blood pressure; HR, heart rate.

### Pathophysiology

The normal physiological response to hypovolaemia is an increase in sympathetic activity to maintain perfusion to the vital organs; heart and brain (Maier, 2005). Hypovolaemia initiates a multi-system response to maintain cardiac output and organ perfusion:

- Cardiovascular system: the sympathetic nervous system is stimulated and heart rate increases, as does peripheral vaso-constriction. Vasoconstriction is an important compensatory mechanism as 60% of circulating blood volume resides in the venous reservoir.
- Neuroendocrine effects: adrenergic discharge and the secretion of vasopressin and angiotensin produce vasoconstriction, movement of fluid from the interstitial space to the vasculature and maintenance of cardiac output. Aldosterone secretion and vasopressin increase sodium and water retention to increase circulating volume. The secretion of adrenaline, cortisol and glucagon increase the extracellular supply of glucose and make energy stores available for cellular metabolism.

- Immunological effects: stimulation of macrophages induces the production of tumour necrosis factor (TNF), which leads to the production of neutrophils, inflammation and activation of the clotting cascade.
- Renal effects: renal blood flow quickly decreases in hypovolaemic shock. This reduction in renal perfusion may lead to acute tubular necrosis (ATN) and renal failure.
- Haemotological effects: when hypovolaemia is not due to red blood cell loss, for example in diarrhoea, blood becomes viscous, which can lead to microvascular thrombosis.
- Neurological effects: blood flow to the brain is kept constant until systolic pressure falls below 70 mmHg, after which cerebral perfusion is reduced and disordered consciousness will ensue.
- Gastrointestinal effects: hypotension causes a reduction in splanchnic blood flow, which may lead to gut ischaemia (Bongard, 2003).

**Causes**

Causes of hypovolaemic shock include:

- trauma,
- gastrointestinal haemorrhage,
- aortic dissection or ruptured aortic aneurysm,
- ectopic pregnancy,
- severe vomiting and diarrhoea,
- burns,
- peritonitis,
- paralytic ileus,
- excessive diuresis, for example diabetes insipidus,
- bowel obstruction.

**Pathogenesis and clinical features**

The signs and symptoms of hypovolaemia will increase with the severity of fluid loss and can be categorised into three distinctive phases.

*Compensatory stage*

- There is an increase in blood pressure and heart rate due to vasoconstrictive effects of adrenaline and noradrenaline.
- Blood flow to the kidneys reduces as the brain and heart receive the greatest supply and urine output may be reduced.

*Progressive stage*

- Metabolic acidosis increases due to an increase in anaerobic metabolism secondary to reduced perfusion.
- Metabolic acidosis causes arteriolar and pre-capillary sphincters to constrict and blood pools in the capillaries. With histamine release this causes leakage of fluid from the vascular space to the interstitial space and an increase in blood viscosity.
- Vasoconstriction further reduces blood flow to the vital organs.

*Refractory stage*

- Vital organs fail and shock is no longer reversible. Death will ensue.

(Source: Collins, 2000)

**Treatment**

Treatment must be aimed at rapid re-expansion of circulating volume along with interventions to control fluid losses (Maier, 2005). Clinical parameters such as the restoration of urine output, decreased heart rate, increased blood pressure and restoration of mental status should be used to determine whether an adequate amount of fluid has been administered (Bongard, 2003). Using the ABCDE approach as detailed in Chapter 1, treatment should be as follows.

- Airway
- Assess the patient following the ABCDE approach described in chapter 1.
- Evaluate MEWS score and contact medical staff/outreach team where necessary (see p. 298).

- ○ Ensure a patent airway and apply high-flow oxygen via a non-rebreathe mask.
- Breathing
  - ○ Ascertain the rate, rhythm and efficacy of breathing, noting any adverse noises.
- Circulation
  - ○ Insert a wide-bore cannula (preferably two).
  - ○ Volume resuscitate with rapid infusion of warmed isotonic fluid (e.g. 0.9% sodium chloride, 20 ml/kg); should restore haemodynamic parameters.
  - ○ Insert a urinary catheter.
  - ○ Initiate continuous ECG, $SpO_2$ measurement and blood-pressure recordings. Record the core temperature.
  - ○ Take blood for urea and electrolytes, full blood count, blood glucose clotting screen; blood group and cross-match (if haemorrhagic); perform arterial blood gas analysis.
  - ○ Transfuse blood if fluid loss is haemorrhagic (universal donor, O rhesus negative in extreme circumstances).
  - ○ Vasopressor and inotrope therapy have limited use in hypovolaemic shock. The focus of management should be upon treating the cause of the hypovolaemia, e.g. surgical intervention if necessary.
- Disability
  - ○ Ascertain the state conscious using AVPU assessment (see Chapter 6).
  - ○ Monitor the conscious level as a response to resuscitation.
- Exposure
  - ○ Examine the patient and assess for obvious signs of blood or fluid loss, intra-abdominal bleeding, etc.
  - ○ Ensure that the patient is kept warm and exposed for a minimal period of time.

### Central venous pressure (CVP) monitoring in shock

The insertion of a CVC can aid in massive fluid resuscitation as fluid is infused via a central, wide-diameter vein that does not collapse and which can facilitate fluid resuscitation.

CVP monitoring can play a part in the management of the patient in shock. CVP reflects right-atrial filling pressure or right-ventricular preload (Druding, 2000) and is dependent on blood volume, vascular tone and cardiac function (Woodrow, 2000). The normal CVP reading is 0–8 mmHg. A low reading indicates hypovolaemia whereas a high CVP value may be due to hyper-volaemia, cardiac failure and pulmonary embolus. Indications for CVC lines include:

- fluid resuscitation,
- drug administration, for example vasopressors,
- parenteral nutrition,
- measurement of CVP,
- poor venous access,
- cardiac pacing.

## CARDIOGENIC SHOCK

Cardiogenic shock is defined as a state of decreased cardiac output, producing inadequate tissue perfusion despite an adequate or excessive circulating volume and is most often the result of an acute myocardial infarction (MI) (Peacock & Weber, 2004).

Cardiogenic shock is the most lethal form of shock and carries an 80–100% mortality rate (Mower-Wade et al., 2001).

### Causes

- Acute MI with over 40% left-ventricular ischaemia (Peacock & Weber, 2004),
- heart failure,
- cardiomyopathy,
- trauma,
- myocarditis.

(Sources: Collins, 2000; Peacock & Weber, 2004)

### Pathogenesis

Cellular dysfunction at the edge of ischaemic myocardium is exacerbated by hypotension. Cell death may activate inflammatory pathways, increase oxidative stress and worsen dysfunction further. Areas of focal necrosis develop throughout the heart leading to further loss of contractile function and hypotension. This hypotension reduces coronary perfusion pressure and myocardial oxygen delivery. If pulmonary oedema develops this worsens the hypoxia and acidosis and further diminishes myocardial contractility. This series of events rapidly leads to irreversible shock. To compensate for a reduced stroke volume the sympathetic nervous system is activated. Heart rate increases and, via the renin–angiotension mechanism, systemic vascular resistance is increased, as is myocardial oxygen consumption.

### Clinical features

- fast weak pulse,
- systolic blood pressure <90 mmHg,
- urine output <30 ml/h,
- cool pale extremities,
- confusion due to poor cerebral perfusion,
- jugular venous distension,
- fine crackles on chest auscultation.

### Treatment

The goal of treatment is to increase myocardial contractility without increasing heart rate, which will increase myocardial oxygen demand and worsen the condition (Maier, 2005).

- Assess the patient using the ABCDE approach as detailed in Chapter 1.
- Evaluate MEWS score, alert medical staff/outreach team if necessary (see p. 298).
- Administer high-flow oxygen with a non-rebreathe mask.
- Establish monitoring of vital signs: ECG, continuous $SpO_2$, blood pressure, respiratory rate and temperature.
- Establish venous access and take bloods for cardiac markers, urea and electrolytes, magnesium, full blood count, blood glucose, arterial blood gas and serum lactate.
- Record a 12-lead ECG.
- Insert a urinary catheter.

- Relieve chest pain with nitroglyceryl (GTN) and morphine.
- Administer inotropic therapy such as levosimenden or dobutamine to increase cardiac contractility, but note that this is contraindicated if systolic blood pressure is <90 mmHg, because of its vasodilatory effects.
- Manipulate preload, after load and contractility to maintain cardiac output and myocardial perfusion.
- Consider thrombolytic therapy if due to acute MI.
- Commence revascularisation by either percutaneous intervention or coronary bypass.
- Intra-aortic balloon counterpulsation (IABP) is required if the condition is refractory to inotropes. IABP increases the diastolic pressure, which augments coronary perfusion. IABP is a rescue therapy prior to revascularisation techniques.
- Invasive ventilation may be necessary.

(Source: Peacock & Weber, 2004)

## OBSTRUCTIVE SHOCK

Obstructive shock results from impaired ventricular filling (decreased preload) that is severe enough to reduce cardiac output (Greenwald, 2004).

### Causes

- cardiac tamponade,
- tension pneumothorax,
- massive pulmonary embolism.

### Cardiac tamponade

(See Chapter 3)

### Tension pneumothorax

Pneumothorax is an accumulation of air in the pleural space that leads to partial or complete lung collapse (Anonymous, 2002). If the air is not released a build-up of pressure in the mediastinum compresses the heart and distorts the vena cava, reducing venous return and cardiac output. Tension pneumothorax is a potentially life-threatening condition (Allibone, 2003)

*Causes*

- traumatic: due to open or closed chest trauma, particularly if patient is an IPPV;
- iatrogenic: caused by procedures such as insertion of a CVC, or thoracic surgery (Allibone, 2003);
- spontaneous: typically in young healthy adults, or associated with underlying lung disease.

*Clinical features*
Whatever the cause of pneumothorax the clinical signs will remain the same:

- acute shortness of breath,
- asymmetric chest movement,
- hyper-resonance or tympany on percussion,
- respiratory distress with characteristic air hunger,
- hypotension,
- tachypnoea,
- mediastinal shift,
- cardiac arrest.

(source: Anonymous, 2002)

*Treatment*
Tension pneumothorax is a medical emergency and the treatment is immediate release of air from the pleural space.

- Assess the patient using the ABCDE approach as detailed in Chapter 1.
- Evaluate MEWS score, alert medical staff/outreach team as necessary (see p. 298).
- Apply high-flow oxygen with a non-rebreathe mask.
- Initiate continuous ECG monitoring, pulse oximetry, and blood-pressure and respiratory-rate measurements.

- Chest X-ray is not required if the patient is in a state of collapse; diagnosis must be made via clinical findings.
- Insert a large-bore cannula into the second intercostal space, mid-clavicular line to relieve pressure (needle decompression).
- Insertion of a chest tube is mandatory following needle decompression (Anonymous, 2002).
- A post-procedure chest X-ray will demonstrate how much the lung has expanded and whether low-pressure suction is required.
- Administer analgesia as necessary.

## Massive pulmonary embolism

Pulmonary embolism is a common, potentially serious disease associated with a mortality rate of 25% if left untreated (McRae & Ginsberg, 2005). It is the first or second most common cause of unexpected death (Feied & Handler, 2006). Pulmonary embolism is a blockage in the pulmonary artery or branch thereof by clots that embolise. Prolonged venous stasis or significant injury to the veins can provoke deep vein thrombosis (DVT) and pulmonary embolism in any person, but increasing evidence suggests that spontaneous DVT and pulmonary embolism are nearly always related to some underlying hypercoagulable state (Feied & Handler, 2006).

### Causes

Pulmonary embolism can arise from DVT anywhere in the body. Fatal pulmonary embolism often results from thrombus that originates in the axillary or subclavian veins or in the veins of the pelvis. Thrombus that forms around indwelling CVCs is also a common cause of fatal pulmonary embolism. Studies suggest that 50% of patients with a thrombus in the upper leg or thigh will have a pulmonary embolism. DVT of the calf is estimated to be the cause of massive pulmonary embolism in one-third of cases (Feied & Handler, 2006).

## Identifiable risk factors

- prior history of DVT or pulmonary embolism,
- recent surgery, in particular pelvic surgery,
- pregnancy,
- underlying malignancy.

## Clinical features

- tachypnoea: respiratory rate >16 breaths/min,
- pleuritic chest pain,
- dyspnoea,
- hypoxaemia, refractory to oxygen therapy,
- apprehension,
- cough,
- jugular venous distension, indicative of acute obstruction to pulmonary blood flow,
- ECG shows sinus tachycardia in 70% of cases and S1, Q3 can be associated. Echocardiography may show some of the clot or acute right ventricular dilation with tricuspid value incompetence.

## Treatment

Treatment focuses on the restoration and maintenance of cardiac output.

- Assess the patient using the ABCDE approach as detailed in Chapter 1.
- Evaluate MEWS score, alert medical staff/outreach team as necessary (see p. 298).
- Apply high-flow oxygen via a non-rebreathe mask.
- Commence monitoring of vital signs.
- Administer a bolus of 500–1000 ml of normal saline to attempt to maintain blood pressure.
- Give vasopressors if there is no response to fluid challenge.
- Administer thrombolytic therapy, for example ateplase, to attempt to dissolve the embolus if the patient remains haemodynamically unstable despite vigorous fluid resuscitation.

## CONCLUSION

Shock is a potentially life-threatening condition (Collins, 2000) and has many different causes and presentations. A successful outcome for the patient in shock is dependent on early recognition and appropriate, often aggressive resuscitation. It is imperative that nurses recognise the many different presentations of shock, understand its pathogenesis and initiate appropriate management in order to improve outcomes.

## REFERENCES

Ahrens, T (2006) Haemodynamics on sepsis. *AACN Advanced Critical Care* **17**(4), 435–45

Allibone, L (2003) Nursing management of chest drains. *Nursing Standard* **12**(17), 45–56

Annane, D, Bellisant, E & Cavaillon, J (2005) Septic shock. *Lancet* **365**(9453), 63–9

Anonymous (2002) Understanding pneumothorax. *Nursing* **32**(11), 74–5

Bench, S (2004) Clinical skills: assessing and treating shock: a nursing perspective. *British Journal of Nursing* **13**(12), 715–21

Bone, RC, Balk, RA, Cerra FB, Dellinger, RP, Fein, AM, Knaus, WA, et al. (1992) Definitions for sepsis and organ failure and guidelines for the use of innovative therapies in sepsis. The ACCP/SCCM Consensus Conference Committee. American College of Chest Physicians/Society of Critical Care Medicine. *Chest* **101**(6), 1644–55

Bongard, FS (2003) Shock and resuscitation. In Bongard, FS & Sue, DY (eds), *Current Critical Care Diagnosis and Treatment*, 2nd edn, pp. 242–67. Lange Medical Books/McGraw-Hill, New York

Bryant, H (2007) Anaphylaxis: recognition, treatment and education. *Emergency Nurse* **15**(2), 24–8

Collins, T (2000) Understanding shock. *Nursing Standard* **14**(49), 35–9

Crusher, R (2004) Anaphylaxis. *Emergency Nurse* **12**(3), 24–31

Das, UN (2006) Can sepsis and other critical illnesses be predicted and prognosticated? *Advances in Sepsis* **5**(2), 52–9

Dellinger, RP, Carlet, JM, Masur, H, Gerlach, H, Calandra, T, Cohen, J, et al. (2004) Surviving sepsis campaign guidelines for management of severe sepsis and septic shock. *Critical Care Medicine* **32**(3), 858–73

DeMarco, CE & MacArthur, RD (2006) The importance of early and appropriate initial antimicrobial therapy. *Advances in Sepsis* **5**(2), 60–1

Druding, MC (2000) Integrating haemodynamic monitoring and physical assessment. *Dimensions of Critical Care Nursing* **19**(4), 25–30

Elliott, D, Aitken, LM & Chaboyer, W (2007) *Critical Care Nursing*. Elsevier, Chatswood, NSW

Eurle, B & Scalea, TM (2004) Neurogenic shock. In Tintinalli, JE, Kelen, GD & Stapczynski, JS (eds), *Emergency Medicine: a Comprehensive Study Guide*, 6th edn, pp. 252–6. McGraw-Hill, Chicago, IL

Evans, C & Tippins, E (2005) Emergency treatment of anaphylaxis. *Accident and Emergency Nursing* **13**, 232–7

Feied, C & Handler, JA (2006) Pulmonary embolism. www. emedicine.com/emerg/topic490.htm (accessed 5 July 2007)

Ferns, T & Chojnacka, I (2003) The causes of anaphylaxis and it's management in adults. *British Journal of Nursing* **12**(17), 1006–12

Finney, A & Rushton, C (2007) Recognition and management of patients with anaphylaxis. *Nursing Standard* **21**(37), 50–7

Fourrier, F (2004) Recombinant human activated protein C in the treatment of severe sepsis: an evidence-based review. *Critical Care Medicine* **32**(11), S534–41

Gilmore, K & Nanyanzi, C (1999) Pharmacology of vasopressors and inotropes. *World Anaesthesia On line*, issue 10. www.nda. ox.ac.uk/wfsa/html/acrobat/update10.pdf (accessed 7 June 2007)

Greenwald, P (2004) Immediate management of shock. In Stone, CK & Humphries, R (eds), *Current Emergency Diagnosis and Treatment*, 5th edn. McGraw-Hill, CT

Hughes, E (2004) Principles of post-operative patient care. *Nursing Standard* **19**(5), 43–51

Jevon, P (2006) An overview of managing anaphylaxis in the community. *Nursing Times* **102**(39), 48–51

Jui, J (2004) Septic shock. In Tintinalli, JE, Kelen, GD & Stapczynski, JS (eds), *Emergency Medicine: A Comprehensive Study Guide*, 6th edn, pp. 231–41. McGraw-Hill, Chicago, IL

King, JE (2007) Sepsis in critical care. *Critical Care Nursing Clinics of America* **19**, 77–86

Kleinpell, RM, Graves, BT & Ackerman, MH (2006) Incidence, pathogenesis and management of sepsis. *AACN Advanced Critical Care* **17**(4), 385–93

Levy, MM, Fink, MP, Marshall, JC, Abraham, E, Angus, D, Cook, D, et al. (2003) 2001 SCCM/ESICM/ACCP/ATS/SIS International sepsis definitions conference. *Critical Care Medicine* **31**(4), 1250–6

Maier, RV (2005) Approach to the patient with shock. In Kasper, DL, Fauci, AS, Longo, DL, Braunwald, E, Hauser, SL & Jameson, JL (eds), *Harrison's Principles of Internal Medicine*, 16th edn, 1600–5. McGraw-Hill, Columbus, OH

McRae, SJ & Ginsberg, JS (2005) The diagnostic evaluation of pulmonary embolism. *American Heart Hospital Journal* **5**(14), 14–20

Mower-Wade, DM, Bartley, MK & Chiari-Allwein, JL (2001) How to respond to shock. *Dimensions of Critical Care Nursing* **20**(2), 22–7

Parrillo, JE (2005) Severe sepsis and therapy with Activated Protein C. *New England Journal of Medicine* **252**(13), 1398–1400

Peacock, WF & Weber, JE (2004) Cardiogenic shock. In Tintinalli, JE, Kelen, GD & Stapczynski, JS (eds), *Emergency Medicine: A Comprehensive Study Guide*, 6th edn. McGraw-Hill, Chicago, IL

Poeze, M, Ramsay, G, Gerlach, H, Rubulotta, F & Levy, M (2004) An international sepsis survey: a study of doctors' knowledge and perception about sepsis. *Critical Care* **8**(6), R409–13

Powers, J & Jacobi, J (2006) Pharmacologic treatment related to severe sepsis. *AACN Advanced Critical Care* **17**(4), 423–32

Resuscitation Council (UK) (2008) *Emergency Treatment of Anaphylactic Reactions*. Guidelines for health care providers. http://www.resus.org.uk/pages/reaction.pdf (accessed May 2008).

Rhodes, A & Bennett, D (2004) Early goal directed therapy: an evidence-based review. *Critical Care Medicine* **32**(11), S448–50

Rivers, E, Nguyen, B, Havstad, S, Ressler, J, et al. (2001) Early goal-directed therapy in the treatment of severe sepsis and septic shock. *New England Journal of Medicine* **345**(19), 1368–78

Robson, W & Newell, J (2005) Assessing, treating and managing patients with sepsis. *Nursing Standard* **19**(50), 56–64

Russell, JA (2006) Management of sepsis. *New England Journal of Medicine* **355**(916), 1699–1713

Sevransky, JE, Nour, S, Susla, GM, Needham, DM, Hollenberg, S & Pronovost, P (2007) Haemodynamic goals in randomized clinical trials in patients with sepsis: a systematic review of the literature. *Critical Care* **11**(3), 1–9

Sheikh, A & Alves, B (2001) Hospital admissions for acute anaphylaxis: time trend study. *British Medical Journal* **320**(7247), 1441–2

Slade, E, Tamber, PS & Vincent, J (2003) The surviving sepsis campaign: raising awareness to reduce mortality. *Critical Care* **7**, 1–2

Smith, G (2005) *Module 8d: Early Recognition/Identification of sepsis.* PGCert/PGDip/MSc in Critical Care. Wales College of Medicine, Cardiff

Swart, S (2007) Acute pericarditis. *AAOHN Journal* **55**(2), 44–6

Vincent, J & Abraham, E (2006) The last 100 years of sepsis. *American Journal of Respiratory and Critical Care Medicine* **173**(3), 256–63

Woodrow, P (2000) *Intensive Care Nursing, a Framework for Practice.* Routledge, London

# 6 | Neurological Emergencies

## Anthony Batson and Christine Thompson

### INTRODUCTION

Neurological disease accounts for approximately 20% of admissions to general hospitals in the UK, an increasing proportion of which are emergencies (Sharief & Anand, 1997). Neurological emergencies can be life-threatening. Altered conscious level can lead to a compromised airway and compromised breathing. Neurological emergencies require prompt effective treatment, together with close monitoring of ABCDE to detect deterioration.

The aim of this chapter is to allow the reader to understand the treatment of neurological emergencies.

### LEARNING OUTCOMES

At the end of this chapter the reader will be able to:

❏ outline neurological assessment,
❏ describe the causes and clinical features of raised intracranial pressure,
❏ discuss the treatment of altered level of consciousness,
❏ discuss the treatment of stroke,
❏ discuss the treatment of meningitis,
❏ discuss the treatment of head injury,
❏ discuss the treatment of seizures.

### NEUROLOGICAL ASSESSMENT

A full neurological assessment involves assessing:

- level of consciousness,
- pupillary function and eye movements,
- motor function,

- vital signs,
- respiratory pattern.

Of these the most important is level of consciousness (Thelan et al., 1998). Two assessment tools commonly used to determine level of consciousness are:

- AVPU scale,
- Glasgow Coma Scale (GCS).

### AVPU scale

The AVPU scale is a simple and rapid assessment of conscious level (Box 6.1) and assesses whether a person is **A**lert, responds only to **V**oice, responds only to **P**ain or is **U**nresponsive to all stimuli and is dependent on the person's eye-opening ability. The AVPU scale is commonly used when rapidly assessing a critically ill patient (the ABCDE approach; see Chapter 1).

A more definitive and widely used tool is the Glasgow Coma Scale (GCS) developed by Teasdale and Jennet in 1974 (Waterhouse, 2005). Although originally designed to assess and monitor patients with acute head injuries, it is now widely recognised as a useful tool for monitoring level of consciousness in any patient with compromised neurological function.

GCS assesses three criteria (eye opening, verbal response and motor response) on a numerical scoring system (Box 6.2). The best response in each category is scored. The fully alert and awake person will score the maximum possible of 15, and the totally

---

**Box 6.1 The AVPU scale**

A = **A**lert
V = Responds to **v**oice (speech)
P = Responds to **p**ainful stimuli
U = **U**nresponsive to any stimulus

Source: Resuscitation Council UK (2006).

---

---

**Box 6.2 Summary of the Glasgow Coma Scale (GCS)**

Best eye-opening response:

- eye opening spontaneously (scores 4),
- eye opening to speech (scores 3),
- eye opening to pain (scores 2),
- no response (scores 1).

Best verbal response:

- orientated (scores 5),
- confused (scores 4),
- inappropriate words (scores 3),
- incomprehensible sounds (scores 2),
- no response (scores 1).

Best motor response:

- obeys commands (scores 6),
- localises pain (scores 5),
- withdraws from pain (scores 4),
- abnormal flexion (scores 3),
- extension (scores 2),
- no response (scores 1).

---

unresponsive person will score the minimum possible of 3; as well as calculating the total GCS score, the score for each individual component (e.g. E2, M4, V4) must be given since this reflects the overall status much more accurately (NICE, 2003).

By assessing and recording the GCS on a regular basis it is possible to monitor the patient's level of consciousness and detect any signs of deterioration. Deterioration by 1 point in motor response and 2 points in the overall GCS score is clinically significant and should be brought to the immediate attention of senior staff (NICE, 2003; Waterhouse, 2005).

It is important to try to ensure consistency of GCS scores recorded by different nurses (Woodrow, 2000). The National Neuroscience Benchmarking Group (2006) suggests that one nurse on each shift should be responsible for checking and recording the neurological observations on the patient, as this will ensure consistency. Consistency would also be assured if at the change-over of shifts the two nurses carried out a set of observations together.

When assessing best eye-opening response, the following points should be noted.

- *Eye opening spontaneously (scores 4)*: when the patient is awake with eyes open. If eyes are closed when you approach the patient, the eyes should open without need for speech or touch (Waterhouse, 2005). If the face is so swollen that it is difficult or impossible to open the eyes, this must be recorded with the letter C.
- *Eye opening to speech (scores 3)*: do not touch the patient but speak in a normal voice. If no response, gradually raise your voice.
- *Eye opening to pain (scores 2)*: first, touch or gently shake the patient's shoulder. If there is no response a deeper stimulus is applied. Waterhouse (2005) suggests that peripheral pressure is appropriate here and should be applied gradually to the lateral outer aspect of the second or third finger (she suggests that only peripheral painful stimuli be applied at this stage of the assessment since the application of a central stimulus produces a grimacing effect and makes patients close their eyes instead of opening them).
- *No response (scores 1)*: the patient's eyes do not open even with persistent verbal or painful stimulation.

Adapted from Dawson and Shah (2003) and Waterhouse (2005).

When assessing best verbal response, the following points should be noted.

- *Orientated (scores 5)*: this assesses the patient's orientation to time, place and person. The patient is able to accurately state the date and where and who he or she is.
- *Confused (scores 4)*: the patient is able to form sentences but is unable to answer all questions correctly.

- *Inappropriate words (scores 3)*: the patient's responses are restricted to words that are recognisable, but inappropriate to the questions asked.
- *Incomprehensible sounds (scores 2)*: the patient makes sounds that are not recognisable as words; these may be limited to cries, moans or groans.
- *No response (scores 1)*: the patient does not make any sounds to any type of stimulus.

Adapted from Dawson and Shah (2003) and Waterhouse (2005).

Best verbal response can be difficult to assess if the patient:

- is not from the locality: they may not know exactly where they are;
- is unable to speak/understand the local language;
- is intubated: this will prevent a verbal response and thus lower the total score, and in this circumstance intubation should be identified by a letter T;
- has dysphasia, which may prevent the patient from giving a coherent response and again will affect the scores. In this instance dysphasia should be represented by a letter D;
- has a spinal injury/paralysis or hearing deficit;
- is under the influence of drugs, for example anaesthetic, or alcohol or illicit drug use;
- Scoring each individual component will give a much more accurate picture.

When assessing best motor response, the following points should be noted.

- *Obeys commands (scores 6)*: the patient can accurately follow simple instructions, such as 'stick your tongue out' or 'squeeze and release my hand'. (It is important that you ask the patient to release your hand since grasping (squeezing) alone may be a simple reflex).
- *Localises pain (scores 5)*: the patient responds to a centrally applied stimulus (Box 6.3) by raising a hand towards the pain source 'in an obvious co-ordinated attempt to remove the cause

---

**Box 6.3 Methods of applying a painful stimulus**

Trapezium squeeze–Squeezing the trapezius muscle between the neck and shoulder.

Supra-orbital pressure–Applying firm pressure with the thumb to the ridge under the eyebrow. This is not recommended if facial fracture is suspected (Hickey, 2003).

Jaw margin pressure–Pressure applied with the flat part of the thumb against the corner of the maxillary and mandibular junction.

---

of the pain' (Waterhouse, 2005). This should be applied only if the patient has not responded to a verbal stimulus.

- *Withdraws from pain (scores 4)*: the patient's arms bend (flex) at the elbow in response to a central painful stimulus, but fail to locate the pain source.
- *Abnormal flexion (scores 3)*: the forearm is flexed and the hand flexes and rotates at the wrist. This is known as decorticate posturing.
- *Extension (scores 2)*: the arms straighten at the elbow, the shoulders and forearms are internally rotated and the wrists are flexed. The legs may be extended with the toes pointing downwards. This is decerebrate posturing.
- *No response (scores 1)*: there is no response from the patient to a deeply painful stimulus.

Adapted from Dawson and Shah (2003) and Waterhouse (2005).

Note: if the patient is receiving paralysing drugs then the letter P must be recorded.

### Assessment of the pupils

Assessment of the pupils is especially important in patients who are sedated when the GCS cannot be relied upon (Cree, 2003).

Indeed, the American College of Surgeons Committee on Trauma (2004) advocate performing GCS and pupillary examination prior to sedation. The nurse has an essential role in assessing pupillary responses as part of the central nervous system (CNS) assessment (Geraghty, 2005).

If the patient's eyes do not open to speech or to pain, it will be necessary to physically lift the eyelids so that the pupils can be assessed. If the eyes are swollen, it may not be possible to do this or doing it may worsen the injury. In these circumstances document C for closed on the chart (Box 6.4).

Assess the pupils for the following features.

- Size: 'normal' pupil size is 2–5 mm (Hickey, 2003). Although often used, the term 'pinpoint' is best avoided as it is subjective and not objective.
- Shape: normally round. If they are not round, try to establish whether there has been previous injury or surgery to explain the abnormal shape.
- Equality: pupils should be equal; sometimes pupils are unequal without any related pathological disorder (Hickey, 2003): try to establish whether this is usual for the patient.
- Reactivity: the room should ideally be slightly darkened or the eyes shaded to dilate the pupils. This will facilitate the assessment of reactivity of the pupils because their constriction, following the shining of a light into each eye, will be more pronounced. Note any pre-existing ophthalmic condition

---

**Box 6.4 Documentation of pupil reactivity**

+ Brisk reaction
− No reaction
s Sluggish reaction: an important finding indicating deterioration
c Eye closed

---

---

**Box 6.5 Assessment of pupils: abnormal findings**

Very small pupils–Possible opioid use

Very large pupils–Possible amphetamine use; mydriatic use

Inequality in size or reaction–May indicate the third cranial nerve (oculomotor) being compressed on the same side (ipsilateral) of the brain as the affected pupil. This is usually as a result of a bleed or other swelling in the brain and this is an emergency (Smith, 2000). A mildly dilated pupil and a sluggish reaction may be an early sign of this (Emergency Nurses Association, 2000).

No reaction–Fixed and dilated pupils suggest an advanced problem possibly indicating irreversible damage, although use of drugs such as atropine, as well as anticholinergic use and seizure activity (Advanced Life Support Group, 2001) need to be considered as a possible causes. 'A widely dilated pupil occasionally occurs with direct trauma to the globe of the eye' (Emergency Nurses Association, 2000; American College of Surgeons Committee on Trauma, 2004).

---

leading to unequal pupils, for example cataract (Waterhouse, 2005). Use a bright light (pen torch), not an ophthalmoscope, as these are designed to visualise the retina and to avoid pupil constriction; and document findings for each eye in turn (see Box 6.4). Observe each pupil for reaction and then test each pupil again, this time observing both the pupils for reactions. The left pupil should also constrict when the right pupil is exposed to light and vice versa. This is called the consensual response. The significance of the findings are detailed in Box 6.5. Changes in pupil reaction and size may be a late sign of raised intracranial pressure (Waterhouse, 2005).

### Vital signs

The patient's vital signs should be monitored regularly. The rate and depth of breathing should be noted carefully and, because respiration is controlled by more than one centre in the brain, this provides important information about cerebral function (Dougherty & Lister, 2004) since pressure on the respiratory centres cause impairment of respiratory patterns (Waterhouse, 2005). Abnormal patterns include Cheyne–Stokes breathing and cluster breathing (for more details see Jevon & Ewens, 2007).

Damage to the temperature-regulating centre in the hypothalamus from either primary or secondary insult can lead to temperature changes, often hyperthermia. Pyrexia increases cerebral oxygen consumption, and reduces cerebral perfusion and therefore cerebral oxygen supply, leading to worsening cerebral ischaemia and damage (Woodrow, 2000).

In a patient with a neurological emergency, hypotension could indicate end-stage cerebral failure or spinal shock (Dawson & Sanders, 2000), although other causes of hypotension, for example hypovolaemia or sepsis, must be sought and addressed. Hypertension (typically with a high systolic pressure but a comparatively unchanged diastolic pressure) can be associated with raised intracranial pressure; that is, the body's response to try to perfuse the brain (Waterhouse, 2005).

Bradycardia is a sign of a cerebral insult; the heart rate slows in an effort for each contraction to pump more blood into the brain at high pressure and achieve cerebral perfusion. This is a late sign (Waterhouse, 2005)

Altered respiratory pattern, hypertension and bradycardia are together termed Cushing's triad or reflex; they are a set of signs indicating raised intracranial pressure and should alert the healthcare professional that the patient is critically ill and at risk of 'coning' (herniation of the brain stem into the foramen magnum) and of death. Once this has occurred, the patient's level of consciousness will have deteriorated (Dougherty & Lister, 2004).

## CAUSES AND CLINICAL FEATURES OF RAISED INTRACRANIAL PRESSURE

Raised intracranial pressure may be a feature of a number of cerebral disorders. The Monro–Kellie hypothesis states that the rigid cranium is filled with three non-compressible substances: brain tissue, cerebrospinal fluid (CSF) and blood (contained in the vessels). The volumes of these remain relatively constant. If the volume of any one increases, then this has to be balanced by a corresponding reduction in the volume of another in order for homeostasis to be maintained. Any increase in one substance without the corresponding decrease in another will increase the intracranial pressure (Hickey, 2003). Causes of raised intracranial pressure include:

- increased CSF,
- intracranial haemorrhage,
- cerebral swelling,
- brain tumour,
- hypoxia,
- hypovolaemia,
- hypercapnia,
- pain,
- turning in bed,
- suction,
- seizures,
- increased intrathoracic pressure.

Clinical features of raised intracranial pressure include:

- headaches,
- altered consciousness,
- nausea and vomiting,
- loss of temperature regulation (may be hypo-/hyperthermic),
- changes in pupillary equality, size, shape and reactivity,
- increasing blood pressure,
- decreasing pulse rate,
- altered respiratory patterns.

(Hickey, 2003)

## ALTERED CONSCIOUS LEVEL

The term coma, which has derived from the Greek meaning 'deep sleep', has traditionally been used quite loosely to describe a wide spectrum of neurological conditions in which the main feature is altered conscious level (Grange & Watson, 1997). There are many causes of altered conscious level (see below); the history of the mode of its onset, together with any precipitating event, are crucial to establish the cause.

### Causes

Causes of altered conscious level include:

- metabolic disturbances, for example hypoglycaemia or hypothyroidism;
- trauma, for example head injury;
- cerebrovascular disease, for example stroke or subarachnoid haemorrhage;
- infections, for example meningitis;
- drugs, for example opiates.

(Boon et al., 2006)

### Investigations

Investigations are mainly aimed at helping diagnosis, for example toxic screen (drug overdose), blood sugar (hypoglycaemia or hyperglycaemia), CT/MRI scan (cerebral insult) and arterial blood gas analysis (hypercapnia).

### Treatment

- Assess the patient following the ABCDE approach described in Chapter 1. Evaluate MEWS score and alert medics/ outreach if necessary (see p. 298).
- Ensure that the patient has a clear airway. The airway can become compromised by the tongue and/or secretions, vomit in the mouth. If the patient is unconscious (but breathing), place in the recovery position (Figure 6.1) and consider inserting an oropharyngeal airway. Regular oral suction may be required. Some patients will require tracheal intubation and positive-pressure ventilation.
- Monitor the patient's airway regularly (Wyatt et al., 2006).
- Administer high-flow oxygen using a non-rebreathe mask (Figure 1.4). Monitor the patient's breathing closely as ventila-

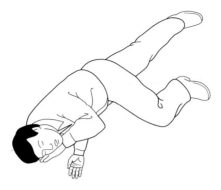

**Figure 6.1** The recovery position

tory support may be required. Establish oxygen-saturation monitoring using a pulse oximeter.

- Insert a wide-bore intravenous (IV) cannula (e.g. 14 gauge) and commence IV fluids to maintain hydration.
- Monitor the patient's vital signs closely. Commence ECG monitoring and record a 12-lead ECG.
- Monitor the patient's level of consciousness closely, using the AVPU and GCS scales; undertake regular assessment of the pupils.
- Perform bedside blood glucose measurement. Correct hypoglycaemia if present; correct hyperglycaemia if present (Hickey, 2003).
- Check the patient's medication chart for recent administration of a mediation that may cause unconsciousness, for example an opiate; administer appropriate antidote if indicated.
- Closely monitor the patient's temperature. Pyrexia increases cerebral metabolic rate which can cause cerebral oedema (Hickey, 2003); prescribed anti-pyretics should be administered if required.
- Insert a urinary catheter and monitor urine output.
- Monitor the patient's pressure areas, particularly if the patient has been incontinent.

- Ensure natural positioning of limbs, hands, digits, particularly on the affected side so as to avoid injury.

## STROKE

A stroke can be defined as a focal or global neurological deficit with symptoms lasting more than 24 h (World Health Organization, 2004; Wyatt et al., 2006). A stroke is a medical emergency (Stroke Association, 2005) requiring immediate treatment, which is directed towards sustaining life and preventing further brain damage.

### Pathogenesis

Although strokes can occur in all age groups, 70% occur in patients over 70 years of age (Wyatt et al., 2006). They are caused by either cerebral infarction or cerebral haemorrhage.

- Cerebral infarction (80%): due to thrombosis, cerebral embolism (e.g. from atrial fibrillation or valve disease/replacement) or very occasionally an episode of hypoperfusion.
- Cererbral haemorrhage (20%): associated with hypertension, subarachnoid haemorrhage and bleeding disorders.

(Wyatt et al., 2006)

### Clinical features

Clinical features will depend on the type of stroke, the area affected and the extent of the stroke. However, these may include:

- weakness or paralysis of one side of the body,
- sudden severe unexplained headache,
- loss of balance,
- loss of sensation in the affected area,
- speech and swallowing difficulty,
- visual problems,
- drooling,
- numbness and tingling in affected areas,
- unconsciousness.

**Investigations**

Routine bloods should be taken including glucose measurement. A 12-lead ECG should be recorded, primarily to detect atrial fibrillation (commonly associated with cerebral embolism). If there is any doubt about the diagnosis or if neurosurgery may benefit the patient, a CT/MRI scan should be requested (Wyatt et al., 2006).

**Treatment**

- Assess the patient following the ABCDE approach described in Chapter 1. Evaluate MEWS score and alert medics/outreach if necessary (see p. 298).
- If the patient is conscious, ensure that the head and shoulders are supported in a slightly raised position to help protect the airway; tilt the head towards the affected side to allow secretions to drain out; wipe the mouth with a flannel or similar.
- Ensure that the patient has a clear airway. Following a stroke the airway can become compromised by the tongue and/or secretions in the mouth. Ensure that the patient's airway remains patent: aspiration of gastric contents or secretions is a serious complication of a stroke, which is associated with considerable morbidity and mortality (American Heart Association, 2000). If the patient is unconscious (but breathing), place in the recovery position and consider inserting an oropharyngeal airway. If the patient is conscious, ensure that the head and shoulders are supported in a slightly raised position, to help protect the airway; tilting the head towards the affected side allows secretions to drain out; wipe the mouth with a flannel or similar (British Red Cross, 2003). Regular oral suction may be required. Some patients will require tracheal intubation and positive-pressure ventilation.
- Monitor the patient's airway regularly and do not give them anything to eat or drink until the ability to swallow has been assessed thoroughly (Wyatt et al., 2006).

- Administer high-flow oxygen using a non-rebreathe mask (Figure 1.4). Closely monitor the patient's breathing as ventilatory support may be required. Establish oxygen-saturation monitoring using a pulse oximeter.
- Insert a wide-bore IV cannula (e.g. 14 gauge) and commence IV fluids to maintain hydration.
- Monitor the patient's vital signs closely. An elevated blood pressure is a normal compensatory mechanism following a stroke (Thelan et al., 1998), although if the stroke has been caused by cerebral haemorrhage, severe hypertension could worsen the damage. However, hypotension can lead to hypoperfusion and cerebral ischaemia; a systolic blood pressure of <100 mmHg and a diastolic blood pressure of <70 mmHg are associated with neurological deterioration, poor outcome and death (Castillo et al., 2004). Therefore if severe hypertension is present, great care should be taken to ensure that efforts to reduce blood pressure are not too aggressive, since this may lead to too severe a fall and a worsening of neurological status (Johnston & Mayer, 2003; Goldstein, 2004). Anti-hypertensive therapy should only be administered under expert advice (Wyatt et al., 2006).
- Minimise factors that could increase the patient's blood pressure, for example recognise and relieve pain, abolish nausea, vomiting and stress; and offer relief from the discomfort of a full bladder (Rees et al., 2002).
- If the cause of the stroke is an infarction (i.e. haemorrhage has been excluded), administer aspirin 300 mg (anti-platelet) as this reduces both morbidity and mortality (Wyatt et al., 2006).
- Closely monitor the patient's level of consciousness, using AVPU and if necessary the GCS scale.
- Perform bedside blood glucose measurement. Correct hypoglycaemia if present; correct hyperglycaemia if present as it may increase the size of the cerebral infarct (Hickey, 2003).
- Closely monitor the patient's temperature. Pyrexia increases cerebral metabolic rate which can cause cerebral oedema

(Hickey, 2003); prescribed anti-pyretics should be administered if required.

- Insert a urinary catheter if the patient has urinary retention or is unconscious (Wyatt et al., 2006); monitor urine output.
- Monitor the patient's pressure areas, particularly if the patient has been incontinent.
- Ensure natural positioning of limbs, hands, digits, etc., particularly on the affected side so as to avoid injury.
- Involve the stroke team at the earliest opportunity. Nursing the patient on a dedicated stroke unit improves outcome (Wyatt et al., 2006).
- Reassure the patient. Once the patient regains consciousness the patient may be disorientated and may have a headache that requires analgesia.

## MENINGITIS

Meningitis can be defined as inflammation of the meninges (Bowler, 1998; National Meningitis Trust, 2003). Although more common in children, it can affect adults (Endacott, 2003). Meningitis can be classified as:

- viral meningitis: the most common form, usually 4–10 days in duration; the patient normally makes a full recovery, although headaches and malaise may persist;
- bacterial meningitis: is the most serious form, since it is life-threatening and is associated with a rapid onset and disease progression;
- fungal meningitis: uncommon, usually affecting the immuno-compromised patient.

(Bowler, 1998; National Meningitis Trust, 2003)

The most common causes of bacterial meningitis are described below.

- *Streptococcus pneumoniae*: the childhood immunisation programme now includes a vaccination against pneumococcus (Department of Health, 2006), which will hopefully reduce incidence.

- *Neisseria menigitidis* (meningococcus): can cause meningococcal septicaemia and is associated with a high mortality rate (5–10% in developed countries) and survivors may be left with persistent neurological defects (approximately 20%) even when effective antibiotic treatment is available (Boyne, 2001). Of the 13 recognised subgroups of this bacteria three are globally important – A, B and C – and of these B and C are significant in the UK. There is an effective vaccination against group C meningococcus which is now included in the UK's childhood immunisation progamme but no vaccine currently exists against group B, the predominant cause of meningococcal infection in the UK (Boyne, 2001) accounting for two-thirds of meningococcal infection (National Meningitis Trust, 2003). The bacterium is 'carried' in the nasopharynx of many healthy individuals; approximately 10% of the general population rising to 25% in those aged 15–19 years carry a strain of the bacterium (National Meningitis Trust, 2003).
- *Haemophilus influenza*: incidence is on the decline since the introduction of the Hib vaccination in the childhood immunisation progamme (Bird & Lorkin, 2000).

**Clinical features**

It can be difficult to detect meningococcal meningitis and septicaemia in the early stages because both can display clinical features similar to influenza (Bowler, 1998; Boyne, 2001). Elderly patients may lack specific symptoms (National Meningitis Trust, 2003).

Clinical features include:

- influenza-type symptoms,
- headache,
- neck stiffness,
- decrease in conscious level,
- skin rash: this occurs in 50% of cases of meningococcal meningitis, usually presenting with a maculopapular rash before the characteristic petechial rash develops.

(Sources: National Meningitis Trust, 2003; Wyatt et al., 2006)

### Investigations

Initial investigations should include full blood count, blood glucose, urea and electrolytes, clotting screen, blood cultures and C-reactive protein; a throat swab should be taken as this will be positive in 40% of meningococcal infections (Wyatt et al., 2006). A lumbar puncture may be performed to confirm diagnosis, but not if there is increased intracranial pressure or coagulopathy (Wyatt et al., 2006).

Meningism (irritation of the meninges) is best elicited by passive flexion of the neck when the patient is supine (Advanced Life Support Group, 2001). This can be confirmed by a positive Kernig's test where the leg is flexed at the hip and the knee gradually extended; resistance to this by contraction of the hamstrings is indicative of meningeal irritation (Advanced Life Support Group, 2001).

### Treatment

- Ensure that local infection control procedures are followed. It may be necessary to nurse the patient in a side-room.
- Assess the patient following the ABCDE approach described in Chapter 1. Evaluate MEWS score and alert medics/outreach if necessary (see p. 298).
- Ensure that the patient has a clear airway. If the patient has altered conscious level, place in the lateral position.
- Administer high-flow oxygen using a non-rebreathe mask (Figure 1.4). Establish oxygen-saturation monitoring using a pulse oximeter. Monitor the patient's breathing closely.
- Insert a wide-bore IV cannula (e.g. 14 or 16 gauge) and commence IV fluids to maintain hydration.
- Monitor the patient's vital signs closely. If the patient is in shock, commence fluid resuscitation intravenously and commence inotropic support in addition. In sepsis, consider activated Protein C following local guidelines.
- Administer prescribed antibiotics, usually cefotaxime 2 g IV four times a day (BNF, 2007).
- Perform bedside blood glucose measurement. Correct hypoglycaemia if present.

- Closely monitor the patient's level of consciousness, using AVPU and if necessary the GCS scale.
- Closely monitor the patient's temperature. Pyrexia increases cerebral metabolic rate which can cause cerebral oedema (Hickey, 2003); prescribed anti-pyretics should be administered if required.
- Administer dexamethasone 0.15 mg/kg IV as indicated (Wyatt et al., 2006).
- If the patient has a headache, administer prescribed analgesia, for example paracetamol 1 g orally.
- If the patient has nausea and vomiting, administer prescribed anti-emetic, for example metoclopramide 10 mg IV.
- Ensure a dark and quiet environment. Avoid bright lights especially if the patient complains of photophobia. Noisy environments will also increase irritability (Muxlow, 2000).
- Meningococcal meningitis is a notifiable disease. Inform the Centre for Communicable Diseases and consider whether the close contacts of the patient require prophylactic antibiotics.

## HEAD INJURIES

Traumatic head injury is a major cause of death and disability in trauma patients (Hickey, 2003). In the UK head injuries account for approximately 1.4 million admissions to emergency departments each year. Of these about 5000 will die (Dolan & Holt, 2000). Some of the major causes of head injuries include motor vehicle accidents, falls, acts of violence and sport-related injuries.

The term head injury generally refers to any injury to the scalp, skull (cranium and facial bones) and/or the brain. However, head injuries that require hospitalisation (even if it is only for a very short duration) suggest an injury which is sufficiently severe to affect normal cerebral function.

Although head injury is considered a surgical condition, medical patients are admitted with associated head injuries, hence the need to include a brief overview to the treatment of head injuries in this chapter.

**Severity of head injuries**

The severity of head injury is classified as:

- mild: GCS 13–14,
- moderate: GCS 9–12,
- severe: GCS 8 or less.

(Dawson & Shah, 2003).

**Classification**

Head injuries can be classified according to the mechanics and location of injury:

- acceleration: caused by an object striking a stationary head;
- deceleration: caused by the head moving to strike a stationary object;
- coup: damage directly under the area of impact;
- contrecoup: damage opposite to the point of impact;
- open: wound to the scalp and cranium, and the cranial contents are exposed;
- closed: no obvious breaks in the skin;
- contusion: bruising and other damage to brain tissue;
- focal: confined to a specific area of the brain;
- diffuse: affecting more than one area of the brain.

(Source: Zink, 2005)

**Description of head injuries**

- Scalp: contusions, lacerations.
- Skull (simple fracture): usually a linear break in the bone without displacement, hence the bone does not pierce the dura or brain. However, there may be contusion to the brain tissue as a result of acceleration/deceleration forces which are a marker of energy transfer. The inner aspects of the cranial bones are grooved, and sitting in the grooves are blood vessels. In addition, with a linear fracture, blood vessels may be torn, causing bleeding between the bone and the dura (extra-dural haemorrhage). The vessel most susceptible to this injury is the middle meningeal artery (Thelan et al., 1998).

- Skull (compound fracture): may be comminuted (where the bone is shattered and damages the underlying structures) and/or depressed (where the bone is pushed into the underlying structures). In addition to damaging the meninges and brain tissue, compound fractures may also be associated with intracranial haemorrhage and risk of infection.
- Basal skull fracture: the fragile bones at the base of the skull are very intimately related to the dura and often the fracture involves tearing of the dura, this will cause leakage of CSF from the ears (otorrhoea) and from the nose (rhinorrhoea) (Hickey, 2003). Ring-like bruising around the eyes ('raccoon's eyes') and bruising behind the ears ('Battle's sign') may also be evident.
- Meninges: may be torn or displaced, especially the dura. Blood vessels may also be torn giving rise to haemorrhage and haematoma formation. Bleeding from torn vessels which occurs between the dura and the cranium is an extra-dural (or epidural) haemorrhage (EDH). Classically most such haemorrhages are arterial in origin (Hickey, 2003) and associated with rapid deterioration following variable periods of lucidity. Bleeding between the dura and arachnoid is a sub-dural haemorrhage (SDH) and may be categorised, according to the interval between the initial trauma and the appearance of symptoms, as acute, sub-acute or chronic. Bleeding between the arachnoid and pia mater (into the sub-arachnoid space) is a sub-arachnoid haemorrhage (SAH). These are less frequently associated with traumatic brain injury, but may occur as a result of damage through shearing forces (Dolan & Holt, 2000). Any bleeding occurring inside the cranium, regardless of its location, will increase the volume of the cranial contents and thus cause increased intracranial pressure.
- Brain tissue – concussion: an immediate and temporary impairment of brain function and may or may not be associated with loss of consciousness.
- Brain tissue – contusion: bruising to the brain tissue due to rupturing of small blood vessels in the brain tissue. When larger blood vessels within the brain tissue rupture and bleed, this is an intracerebral haemorrhage.

- Cerebral oedema: swelling of the brain tissue following trauma.
- Haematoma: may be epidural (extra-dural), sub-dural, sub-arachnoid or intracerebral.

### Outcomes following head injury

Outcomes following a head injury are dependent upon the following.

- Primary brain injury: that is, damage resulting from the initial impact. It is generally acknowledged that primary damage is irreversible.
- Secondary brain injury: that is, damage which occurs as a result of the initial injury and may occur at any time following the initial injury, for example haemorrhage and haematoma formation, brain swelling, cerebral ischaemia, cerebral hypoxia, raised intracranial pressure or infection. Secondary brain injury may be preventable or reversible (Hickey, 2003; Zink, 2005), and any subsequent deterioration is due to secondary and potentially preventable causes, the most common being hypoxia and hypovolaemia, both of which contribute to raised intracranial pressure, a major cause of death in head injury.

### Treatment of severe head injury

- Assess the patient following the ABCDE approach described in Chapter 1. Evaluate MEWS score and alert medics/outreach if necessary (see p. 298).
- Ensure that the patient has a clear airway. The airway can become compromised by the tongue and/or secretions, vomit, blood in the mouth. Oral suction may be required; care should be taken to avoid hypoxaemia and raised intracranial pressure (Bahouth & Yarbrough, 2005). If the patient is unconscious (but breathing), place in the recovery position (Figure 6.1) and consider inserting an oropharyngeal airway (caution if the patient has a suspected cervical spine injury).
- Regularly monitor the patient's airway (Wyatt et al., 2006).

- Administer high-flow oxygen using a non-rebreathe mask (Figure 1.4). Establish oxygen-saturation monitoring using a pulse oximeter. Monitor the patient's breathing closely as ventilatory support may be required.
- Insert a wide-bore IV cannula (e.g. 14 gauge). A blood sample for routine blood should be taken. In addition, group and save/cross-match may be required. It may be necessary to commence IV fluids to maintain hydration. If shock is present, start fluid resuscitation; blood transfusion may be indicated.
- Monitor the patient's vital signs closely. Commence ECG monitoring and record a 12-lead ECG.
- Closely monitor the patient's level of consciousness, using AVPU and the GCS scale. If the GCS is less than 9 then tracheal intubation is indicated (Smith, 2000; Hickey, 2003). Undertake regular assessment of the pupils
- Perform bedside blood glucose measurement to exclude hypoglycaemia as a cause of altered conscious level. Both hypoglycaemia and hyperglycaemia may occur following head injury and both contribute to further brain damage (Woodrow, 2000).
- If necessary, administer prescribed analgesia, for example fentanyl or morphine to relieve pain, discomfort and agitation, and to limit response to noxious stimuli, for example suctioning (Bahouth & Yarborough, 2005). Note that opiates cause respiratory depression.
- Closely monitor the patient's temperature. Pyrexia increases cerebral metabolic rate which can cause cerebral oedema (Hickey, 2003); prescribed anti-pyretics should be administered if required.
- Remove clothing and perform a head-to-toe examination of the patient to identify any further injuries and determine appropriate and further investigations and treatment for these (American College of Surgeons Committee on Trauma, 2004).
- If necessary, insert a urinary catheter and monitor urine output
- Provide wound care and tetanus prophylaxis if necessary.
- If necessary, involve the surgical/neurosurgical team; they can provide additional advice on treatment, as well as on the possible need for surgical intervention (Driscoll et al., 1993).

## SEIZURES

Seizures (convulsions or fits) consist of involuntary muscle contractions. There are in excess of 40 different types of seizure (Epilepsy Action, 2004) and approximately 2–10% of the population will experience a seizure at some time in their life (NICE, 2002). Epilepsy is the commonest cause of seizures.

Although seizures are rarely fatal, injuries that can be sustained include fractures, burns, dislocations, concussion and intracerebral haemorrhage (American Heart Association, 2000). Dental injuries are quite common. Maintaining the patient's safety during a seizure is a priority.

The aim of treatment is to halt seizures and prevent irreversible cerebral, systemic, metabolic, autonomic and cardiovascular changes (Shorvon, 2000). Status epilepticus is life-threatening and requires urgent treatment.

### Causes

Causes of seizures include:

- epilepsy (most common cause),
- head injury,
- certain poisons, for example alcohol and ecstasy,
- cerebral hypoxia,
- cerebral hypoglycaemia.

(Jevon, 2006)

### Epilepsy

Epilepsy is a neurological disorder characterised by recurring seizures (Tatum et al., 2004), which are brief and usually characterised by a stereotyped disturbance of consciousness, behaviour, emotion, motor function or sensation resulting from abnormal cortical neuronal discharge (Brown et al., 1998). The external manifestation of the seizure will depend on the part of the brain involved in the neuronal discharge (Hayes, 2004).

Epilepsy affects 430–1000 people per 100,000 (Cockerell et al., 1994). In the UK, 440,000 (1:133) have epilepsy, making it the second most common neurological condition after migraine

(Epilepsy Action, 2004). The majority of individuals (70–85%) with active epilepsy can satisfactorily control recurrent seizures with anti-epileptic drugs (Cilcot et al., 1999).

Sudden unexpected death associated with epilepsy is the principal cause of seizure-related death in people with chronic epilepsy, accounting for approximately 500 deaths each year (NICE, 2002). Although it is not clear what causes these deaths, the most-important risk factor is the frequency of seizures: the more frequent the seizure, the higher the risk. It is estimated that 59% of child deaths and 39% of adult deaths associated with epilepsy could be potentially or probably avoidable (NICE, 2002).

Status epileptics is defined as either a single seizure lasting for 30 min or repeated seizures between which there is incomplete recovery of consciousness; seizures lasting more than 5 min may indicate impending status epilepticus which could be prevented by immediate treatment (Advanced Life Support Group, 2001). Status epilepticus, a potentially life-threatening medical emergency, is associated with significant morbidity and mortality if not treated promptly (NICE, 2003).

### Tonic-clonic seizures

A tonic-clonic seizure, formally termed grand mal fit, is usually characterised by:

- sudden loss of consciousness (often preceded by crying out) and collapse;
- rigidity and arching of the back;
- convulsive movements;
- cyanosis around the mouth (due to irregular respirations);
- clenching of the jaw; saliva may appear at the mouth (could be blood-stained if the casualty has bitten their tongue or lip).

The convulsive movements should stop after a minute, with consciousness gradually returning (the patient usually feels tired and may fall asleep). The casualty may be feel dazed and confused after the event (sources: St John's Ambulance, St Andrew's Ambulance, British Red Cross, 2006; Epilepsy Action, 2004; Jevon, 2006).

## Treatment

- Request help from colleagues.
- Ensure that the environment is safe and protect the patient from injury; ensure that there is space around the patient and remove any potentially dangerous objects, for example hot drinks, from the area if there is a risk of injury (Epilepsy Action, 2004).
- If necessary, cushion the patient's head: place a pillow underneath the patient's head to prevent injury.
- Note the time to check how long the seizure is lasting.
- Carefully observe the patient during seizures (Box 6.6) as a clear history is helpful and is the mainstay of diagnosis (Scottish Intercollegiate Guidelines Network, 2003).

---

**Box 6.6 Routine observations that should be made in a patient having a seizure**

- Where were the patient and what were they doing prior to the seizure?
- Any mood change, e.g. excitement, anger or anxiety?
- Unusual sensations, e.g. odd smell or taste?
- Any prior warning?
- Loss of consciousness or confusion?
- Any colour change, e.g. pallor, cyanosis? If so where, e.g. face, lips, hand?
- Altered respiratory pattern, e.g. dyspnoea, noisy respirations?
- Which part of the body was affected by seizure?
- Incontinence?
- Tongue biting?
- Did the patient do anything unusual, e.g. mumble, wander about or fumble with clothing?
- How long did the seizure last?
- How was the patient following the seizure? Did the patient need to sleep and, if so, for how long?
- How long before the patient can perform normal activities again?

Source: National Society for Epilepsy (2004).

---

- Do not restrain the patient, put anything into the mouth or try to move the patient unless in danger (Epilepsy Action, 2004; National Society for Epilepsy, 2004).
- Once the seizure has stopped, assess the patient following the ABCDE approach described in Chapter 1. Evaluate MEWS score and alert medics/outreach if necessary (see p. 298).
- Ensure that the patient has a clear airway: following a seizure, the patient will have altered conscious level and the airway is at risk. Check the mouth for any injuries and bleeding; suction the mouth if necessary and wipe away any saliva. If the patient is breathing, place in the lateral position and consider inserting a basic airway device, for example oropharyngeal airway; if unable to tolerate oropharyngeal airway consider inserting a nasopharyngeal airway.
- Administer high-flow oxygen using a non-rebreathe mask (Figure 1.4). Establish oxygen-saturation monitoring using a pulse oximeter.
- Insert a wide-bore IV cannula (e.g. 14 or 16 gauge).
- Monitor the patient's vital signs closely.
- Closely monitor the patient's level of consciousness, using AVPU and if necessary the GCS scale.
- Perform bedside blood glucose measurement and correct hypoglycaemia if present; hypoglycaemia can be the cause of a seizure.
- Administer prescribed anti-epileptic medication. Lorazepam 0.1 mg/kg IV (usually a 4-mg bolus) is recommended initially, which can be repeated after 10–20 min if necessary (NICE, 2004). If lorazepam is ineffective at controlling the seizures, phenytoin 18 mg/kg IV over 20 min is recommended (NICE, 2004).
- If IV access is not available, rectal diazepam (first choice) or buccal midazolam (second choice) are alternative options (NICE, 2004), although the latter is not licensed for this use (British National Formulary, 2007).
- As anti-epileptic drugs can cause respiratory depression, closely monitor the patient's respiratory rate and level of con-

sciousness. Lorazepam causes less respiratory depression than diazepam (Morgan, 2001).

- Examine the scalp and face for any injuries. Look for purpura in case of meningococcal infection. History of seizure activity and of past medical events must be taken, especial note needs to be paid to any alcohol abuse, in which case IV thiamine may need to be administered (Advanced Life Support Group, 2001; NICE, 2004)
- Monitor the patient's pressure areas, particularly if the patient has been incontinent.
- If indicated, involve the epilepsy team at the earliest opportunity. Appropriate on-going care is essential.
- If indicated, arrange for appropriate referral to the epilepsy nurse specialist.
- Reassure the patient. Once the patient regains consciousness the patient may be disorientated and may have a headache that requires analgesia.
- Ensure the casualty's head and shoulders are supported in a slightly raised position, to help protect the airway.
- Consider tilting the patient's head towards the weaker side, thus allowing secretions to drain out; wipe the mouth with a flannel or similar (British Red Cross, 2003). Ensure that the casualty's airway remains patent: aspiration of gastric contents or secretions is a serious complication associated with considerable morbidity and mortality (American Heart Association, 2000).
- Do not give the casualty anything to eat or drink.
- Regularly monitor vital signs, particularly the patency of the airway.
- If unconscious, place the casualty in the recovery position.
- Remember wound care and tetanus prophylaxis for any injuries sustained during the seizure.

## SUMMARY

In this chapter neurological assessment, together with the causes and clinical features of raised intracranial pressure, have been discussed. The treatment of common neurological emergencies has been outlined. All patients with a neurological emergency require particularly close monitoring of ABCDE; the airway in particular is at risk if the patient has decreased conscious level.

## REFERENCES

Advanced Life Support Group (2001) *Acute Medical Emergencies. The Practical Approach*, pp. 152, 180. BMJ Publishing, London

American College of Surgeons Committee on Trauma (2004) *Advanced Trauma Life Support for Doctors. Student Course Manual*, 7th edn, pp. 163–4. American College of Surgeons, Chicago, IL

American Heart Association (2000) Guidelines 2000 for cardiopulmonary resuscitation and emergency cardiovascular care – an international consensus on science. *Resuscitation* **46**, 1–448

Bahouth, MN & Yarbrough, KL (2005) Patient management: nervous system. In Morton, PG, Fontaine, DK, Hudak, CM & Gallo, BM (eds), *Critical Care Nursing – a Holistic Approach*, 8th edn, pp. 775–95. Lippincott Williams & Wilkins, Philadelphia, PA

Bird, C & Lorkin, L (2000) Infants. In Dolan, B & Holt, L (eds), *Accident and Emergency Theory into Practice*, pp. 225–48. Balliere Tindall, Edinburgh

Boon, N, Colledge, N & Walker, B (2006) *Davidson's Principles and Practice of Medicine*, 20th edn. Elsevier, Edinburgh

Bowler, S (1998) Meningococcal disease. *Nursing Standard* **13**(5), 49–54

Boyne, L (2001) Meningococcal infection. *Nursing Standard* **16**(7), 47–55

British National Formulary (2007) *British National Formulary*. www.bnf.org.uk/bnf/bnf/53/3617.htm (accessed 10 May 2007). British Medical Association and Royal Pharmaceutical Society of Great Britain, London

British Red Cross (2003) *Practical First Aid*. Dorling Kindersley, Middlesex

Brown, S, Betts, T, Crawford, P, et al. (1998) Epilepsy needs revisited: a revised epilepsy needs document for the UK. *Seizure* **7**, 435–46

Castillo, J, Leira, R, Garcia, MM, Serena, J, Blanco, M & Davalos, A (2004) Blood pressure decrease during the acute phase of ischaemic stroke is associated with brain injury and poor stroke outcome. *Stroke* **35**, 520–6

Cilcot, J, Howell, S, Kemeney, A, et al. (1999) *The Effectiveness of Surgery in the Management of Epilepsy*. Guidance Note for Purchasers InterDec Report 15/1999. Trent Institute for Health Services Research

Cockerell, OC, Hart, YM, Sander, JWAS, et al. (1994) The cost of epilepsy in the United Kingdom: an estimation based on the results of two population based studies. *Epilepsy Research* 18, 249–60

Cree, C (2003) Acquired brain injury: acute management. *Nursing Standard* **18**(11), 45

Dawson, D & Shah, S (2003) Neurological care. In Sheppard, M & Wright, M (eds), *Principles and Practice of High Dependency Nursing*, pp. 159–209. Bailliere Tindall, London

Dawson, D & Sanders, K (2000) Head injuries. In Dolan, B & Holt, L (eds), *Accident and Emergency. Theory into Practice*, pp. 45–65. Balliere Tindall, Edinburgh

Department of Health (2006) *NHS Immunisation Information*. www.immunisation.nhs.uk/hottopic.php?id=23 (accessed 13 June 2007)

Dolan, B & Holt, L (eds) (2000) *Accident and Emergency – Theory into Practice*. Bailliere Tindall, London

Dougherty, L & Lister, S (eds) (2004) *The Royal Marsden Hospital Manual of Clinical Nursing Procedures*, 6th edn, pp. 489–90, 493. Blackwell Publishing, London

Driscoll, PA, Gwinnutt, CL, LeDuc Jimmerson, C & Goodall, O (1993) *Trauma Resuscitation. The Team Approach*, pp. 190–2. Macmillan Press, London

Emergency Nurses Association (2000) *Trauma Nursing Core Course. Provider Manual*, 5th edn, p. 103. Emergency Nurses Association, Des Plaines, IL

Endacott, R (2003) Emergency care of the adult. In Jones, G, Endacott, R & Crouch, R (eds), *Emergency Nursing Care Principles and Practice*, pp. 63–4. Greenwich Medical Media, London

Epilepsy Action (2004) *Epilepsy Information: First Aid For Seizures.* www.epilespy.org.uk (accessed 21 January 2008)

Geraghty, M (2005) Nursing the unconscious patient. *Nursing Standard* **20**(1), 54–64

Goldstein, LB (2004) Blood pressure management in patients with acute ischaemic stroke. *Hypertension* 43, 137–41

Grange, C & Watson, D (1997) Coma: initial assessment and management. In Skinner, D, Swain, A, Robertson, C & Peyton, W (eds), *Cambridge Textbook of Accident and Emergency Medicine*, pp. 167–82. Cambridge University Press, Cambridge

Hayes, C (2004) Clinical skills: practical guide for managing adults with epilepsy. *British Journal of Nursing* **13**(7), 380–6

Hickey, JV (2003) *The Clinical Practice of Neurological and Neurosurgical Nursing*, 5th edn. Lippincott Williams & Wilkins, Philadelphia, PA

Jevon, P (2006) *Emergency Care and First Aid for Nurses.* Elsevier, Oxford

Jevon, P & Ewens, B (2007) *Monitoring the Critically Ill Patient*, 2nd edn. Blackwell Publishing, Oxford

Johnston, KC & Mayer, SA (2003) Blood pressure reduction in ischaemic stroke: a two-edged sword? *Neurology* **61**, 1030–1

Morgan, S (2001) The use of Lorazepam in status epilepticus. *Emergency Nurse* **9**(6), 15–19

Muxlow, J (2000) Caring for the neurological system. In Bassett, C & Makin, L (eds), *Caring for the Seriously Ill Patient*, pp. 146–7. Arnold, London

National Meningitis Trust (2003) *Meningitis Resource Pack*, pp. 7–15, 23–6. www.meningitis-trust.org (accessed 3 May 2007)

National Neuroscience Benchmarking Group (2006) *Neurological Assessment.* British Association of Neuroscience Nurses, North West

National Society for Epilepsy (2004) *Epilepsy: What to do When Someone has a Seizure.* National Society for Epilepsy, Bucks

NICE (2002) NICE launches National Clinical audit of epilepsy-related death. Press release: 2002/026. www.nice.org.uk (accessed 21 January 2008)

NICE (2003) *Head Injury: Triage, Assessment, Investigation and Early Management of Head Injury in Infants, Children and Adults.* Clinical Guideline 4. NICE, London

NICE (2004) *The Epilepsies: Diagnosis and Management of the Epilepsies in Adults in Primary and Secondary Care. Appendix C. Guidelines for Treating Status Epilepticus in Adults and Children.* www.nice.org.uk/nicemedia/pdf/CG020fullguideline_appendixC_corrected.pdf (accessed 21 February 2008)

Rees, G, Shah, S & Handley, C (2002) Subarachnoid haemorrhage: a clinical overview. *Nursing Standard* **16**(42), 47–54

Resuscitation Council UK (2006) *Advanced Life Support Provider Manual*, 5th edn. Resuscitation Council UK, London

Scottish Intercollegiate Guidelines Network (2003) *Diagnosis and Management of Epilepsy in Adults.* Scottish Intercollegiate Guidelines Network, Edinburgh

Sharief, N & Anand, P (1997) Neurological emergencies. In Skinner, D, Swain, A, Robertson, C & Peyton, W (eds), *Cambridge Textbook of Accident and Emergency Medicine*, pp. 1057–77. Cambridge University Press, Cambridge

Shorvon, S (2000) *Handbook of Epilepsy Treatment.* Blackwell, Oxford

Smith, G (2000) *ALERT Acute Life-threatening Events – Recognition and Treatment*, p. 38. University of Portsmouth, Portsmouth

St John's Ambulance, St Andrew's Ambulance, British Red Cross (2006) *First Aid Manual*, 8th edn. Dorling Kindersley, London

Stroke Association (2005) *Stroke is a Medical Emergency.* www.stroke.org.uk/campaigns/current_campaigns/stroke_is_a_medical_emergency/the_emergency.html (accessed 16 May 2007)

Tatum, W, Liporace, J, Benbadis, S & Kaplan, P (2004) Updates on the treatment of epilepsy in women. *Archives of Internal Medicine* **164**(2), 137–45

Teasdale, G & Jennet, B (1974) Assessment of coma and impaired consciousness. A practical scale. *Lancet* **2**, 81–4

Thelan, LA, Urden, LD, Lough, ME & Stacy, KM (eds) (1998) *Critical Care Nursing – Diagnosis and Management*. Mosby, St Louis, MO

Waterhouse, C (2005) The Glasgow Coma Scale and other neurological observations. *Nursing Standard* **19**(33), 56–64

Woodrow, P (2000) Head injuries: acute care. *Nursing Standard* **14**(35), 37–44

World Health Organization (2004) *Deaths by Cause, Sex and Mortality Stratum in WHO Regions, Estimates for 2002*. WHO Report, Annex Table 2. World Health Organization, Geneva

Wyatt, J, Illingworth, R, Graham, C, Clancy, M & Robertson, C (2006) *Oxford Handbook of Emergency Medicine*, 3rd edn. Oxford University Press, Oxford

Zink, E (2005) Head injury. In Morton, PG, Fontaine, DK, Hudak, CM & Gallo, BM (eds), *Critical Care Nursing – a Holistic Approach*, 8th edn, pp. 839–60. Lippincott Williams & Wilkins, Philadelphia, PA

# Acute Renal Failure

# 7

## Sue Talbot

## INTRODUCTION

Acute renal failure (ARF) can be defined as 'an abrupt and sustained decrease in glomerular filtration, urine output or both' (Bellomo et al., 2004). It is a common medical emergency with a significant mortality. In developed countries at least 50% of cases of ARF develop in hospital and are potentially preventable (Armitage & Tomson, 2003).

ARF is characterised by a sudden decline in renal function over hours or days. It can occur in people with previously normal kidney function or underlying kidney disease (Department of Health, 2005) and often requires emergency treatment in the form of renal replacement therapy (RRT). ARF can occur with single-organ failure, with the majority of patients treated on renal wards or high-dependency units, or with multi-organ failure, in which case patients are nursed on critical care units (Royal College of Physicians and Renal Association, 2007).

The aim of this chapter is to allow the reader to understand the management of ARF.

## LEARNING OUTCOMES

At the end of this chapter the reader will be able to:

❏ discuss the incidence of acute renal failure (ARF),
❏ outline the pathophysiology of ARF,
❏ discuss the classification of ARF,
❏ state the specific phases of ARF,
❏ state the clinical and biochemical features associated with ARF,

❏ outline the management of specific problems associated with ARF,

❏ outline renal replacement therapy (RRT).

## INCIDENCE OF ACUTE RENAL FAILURE (ARF)

The numbers of people developing ARF ranges from 172 cases per million of the population to 545 per million of the population, depending on the source (Feest et al., 1993; Stevens et al., 2001; Metcalfe et al., 2002; Robertson et al., 2002). Estimates of the annual incidence of ARF in patients with a creatinine level of >300 μmol/l ranges from 486 per million of the population (Stevens et al., 2001) to 620 per million of the population (Metcalfe et al., 2002). Numbers of those with advanced ARF with a creatinine level of >500 μmol/l ranges between 102 and 140 per million of the population (Metcalfe et al., 2002).

The number of people developing ARF has risen sharply over the last 15 years due to an increasingly elderly population, increased prevalence of chronic kidney disease, and improved survival rates in ischaemic heart disease and diabetes mellitus (Hegarty et al., 2005). The development of ARF in the hospital setting continues to be associated with poor outcomes (Mehta & Chertow, 2003), with one in 20 medical/surgical patients developing ARF (Singri et al., 2003).

## PATHOPHYSIOLOGY OF ARF

Patients at risk of developing ARF are those with sepsis as a precipitating factor (Lamiere et al., 2005), drug induced, underlying chronic kidney disease and older people with cardiovascular disease (Hilton, 2006). Attempts have been made to identify which patients are likely to develop ARF by using the Cleveland Clinic Foundation ARF score (Paganini et al., 1996), but it is still difficult and erratic to predict.

The mortality rate for ARF depends upon the underlying cause but ranges from 40 to 70% (Fry & Farrington, 2006; Hilton, 2006). Thirty per cent of all critically ill patients will develop ARF (Galley, 2000), and the loss of renal function in these patients leads to

---

**Box 7.1 Acute Dialysis Quality Initiative ARF classification**

**R**isk: serum creatinine increased by 1.5 times or decrease in GFR by 25%

**I**njury: serum creatinine increased by 2.0 times or decrease in GFR by 50%

**F**ailure: serum creatinine increased by 3.0 times or decrease in GFR by 75%

**L**oss: persistent ARF, defined as a need for RRT for >4 weeks

**E**nd-stage kidney disease: defined as a need for dialysis for >3 months

Source: Bellomo et al. (2004).

---

increased morbidity and a mortality rate of 65%, with 70% requiring renal replacement therapy (RRT) (McCulloch et al., 1997). Fifty per cent of all patients who develop ARF will die within 90 days, almost always from the primary condition (Metcalfe et al., 2002). In intensive care units 35–50% of ARF cases can be attributed to sepsis (Lamiere et al., 2005), with toxins or ischaemic insult giving a 50–80% mortality rate (Esson & Schrier, 2002). Mortality prediction scores have been used, such as the Acute Physiology and Chronic Health Evaluation score (APACHE III) (Chen et al., 2002), to help identify potential patients who are at risk of developing ARF.

The so-called RIFLE system for ARF (Box 7.1) has been devised, identifying three categories of severity (risk, injury and failure) with an increasing risk for the need for RRT, and two clinical outcomes (loss and end-stage) (Block & Schoolwerth, 2006). This system takes into account glomerular filtration rate (GFR) and urine output.

## CLASSIFICATION OF ARF

ARF can be classified into three categories, as listed below.

- Pre-renal failure (hypoperfusion): decreased renal blood flow, but GFR and tubular function remain normal (40–70% of cases).

- Intrinsic renal failure: direct parenchymal damage associated with the release of renal afferent arteriole vasoconstrictors (10–50% of cases).
- Post renal failure (obstructive): obstructed urine flow by intrinsic or extrinsic masses causes an increase in tubular pressure which decreases GFR. The pressure gradient equalises and maintenance of a depressed GFR is then dependent upon renal afferent vasoconstriction (10% of cases).

(Lamiere et al., 2005; Fry & Farrington, 2006; Hilton, 2006)

**Pre-renal failure**

Pre-renal failure is caused by a true hypovolaemia or a reduction in effective circulating volume such as low cardiac output, systemic vasodilatation or intrarenal vasoconstriction (Box 7.2) (Lamiere et al., 2005) and is the most commonest cause of ARF in hospitals (Fry & Farrington, 2006). The kidney responds to changes in renal perfusion pressure by autoregulation of blood flow and GFR. Renal autoregulation depends upon pre-glomerular vasodilation mediated by prostaglandins, nitric oxide and post-glomerular vasoconstriction mediated by angiotensin II, so they remain fairly constant across a range of mean arterial

---

**Box 7.2 Causes of pre-renal failure**

Volume depletion caused by:

- vomiting,
- diarrhoea,
- burns,
- inappropriate diuresis.

Renal artery stenosis
Hypotension:

- cardiogenic shock,
- sepsis,
- anaphylaxis.

---

pressures (Hilton, 2006). If the mean arterial pressure falls below 70 mmHg autoregulation becomes impaired and leads to ineffective perfusion of the kidneys, leading to a reversible increase in serum creatinine and urea concentration (Lamiere et al., 2005). Urine osmolarity is high and urinary sodium remains low (Armstrong & Bircher, 2002). The structure of the kidneys remains normal.

Some drugs can alter autoregulation and GFR by interfering with the mediators:

- non-steroidal anti-inflammatory drugs (NSAIDs),
- cyclo-oxygenase inhibitors (COX-2 inhibitors),
- angiotensin-converting enzyme inhibitors (ACEIs),
- angiotensin-receptor blockers (ARBs),
- diuretics,
- radiological contrast agents.
    (Lamiere et al., 2005; Fry & Farrington, 2006; Hilton, 2006)

### Intrinsic renal failure

Intrinsic renal failure is associated with structural damage to vessels, glomeruli and renal tubules which is attributed to prolonged or inadequately corrected pre-renal failure (Armitage & Tomson, 2003). The most common cause in hospitals is acute tubular necrosis (Esson & Schrier, 2002) induced by ischaemia, sepsis or toxins and occurs when the reduction in renal blood flow leads to cell necrosis (Singri et al., 2003), although this is rarely seen (Armitage & Tomson, 2003). It is characterised by a sudden decline in the GFR, accumulation of urea and the inability of the kidney to regulate sodium, electrolytes, acids and water. According to Esson and Schrier (2002) there are no uniform diagnostic criteria for acute tubular necrosis, it can be of a lengthy duration and it may lead to ischaemia or cell death. Sinert and Peacock (2006) state that patients can be divided into those with glomerular or tubular aetiologies of renal failure, whereas Hilton (2006) also adds interstitium and vasculature. Causes of acute intrinsic renal failure are listed in Table 7.1.

**Table 7.1** Causes of acute intrinsic renal failure

| Type | Cause |
|------|-------|
| Glomerular disease | Inflammatory: post-infectious glomerulonephritis, Henoch–Schonlein purpura, systemic lupus erythematous<br>Thrombotic: disseminated intravascular coagulation<br>Acute glomerulonephritis |
| Interstitial nephritis | Drug-induced: non-steroidal anti-inflammatory drugs (NSAIDs) and salicylates, antibiotics, anti-convulsants, anti-ulcer agents<br>Granulomatous: sarcoidosis, tuberculosis<br>Infection-related: post-infective, pyelonephritis<br>Auto-immune diseases: systemic lupus erythematous (SLE) |
| Tubular injury | Ischaemia: prolonged renal hypoperfusion secondary to cardiac arrest, haemorrhage, sepsis, drug overdose or surgery<br>Toxins: drugs, e.g. aminoglycosides, radiocontrast media, heavy metals, cisplatinum,<br>Crystals: urate, oxalate<br>Metabolic: hypercalcaemia |
| Vascular | Vasculitis<br>Cryoglobulinaemia<br>Polyarteritis nodosa<br>Thrombitic microangiopathy<br>Cholesterol emboli<br>Renal artery or renal vein thrombosis<br>Hypertensive crisis |

Adapted from Hilton (2006).

**Post renal failure**

Obstructive nephropathy can occasionally present as sub-acute renal failure (Armitage & Tomson, 2003). This must be recognised quickly and a diagnosis made. A prompt intervention such as catheterisation, stenting or a nephrostomy tube (Bennett-Jones, 2006) can result in an improvement or complete recovery of renal function (Fry & Farrington, 2006).

Increased pressure within the renal collecting systems results in a fall in the GFR, reduced tubular reabsorption of sodium and water, acquired tubular acidosis and phosphaturia (Armitage & Tomson, 2003). Other abnormalities of renal tubular function may persist after removal of the obstruction, tubulo-interstitial inflam-

---

**Box 7.3 Intrinsic and extrinsic factors causing post renal failure**

| Intrinsic factors | Extrinsic factors |
| --- | --- |
| Blood clots | Enlarged prostate gland |
| Calculi | Tumours |
| Tumours | Pregnancy |
| Strictures | Aortic aneurysm |
| Drugs, especially those that form crystals, e.g. sulphonamides, acyclovir | Ovarian cysts |
| | Previous gynaecological surgery |

---

mation caused by infiltrating macrophages and T lymphocytes followed by fibrosis, leading to incomplete renal recovery if the obstruction is not removed quickly.

Following removal of the obstruction a profuse diuresis can occur, with 4–20 litres being reported over a 24-h period. It only occurs following obstruction of both kidneys or a single functioning kidney and can lead to patients becoming volume depleted. Therefore, careful monitoring and adjustment of volume and electrolyte status is needed. The causes of post renal failure can be classified into intrinsic and extrinsic factors (Box 7.3).

SPECIFIC PHASES OF ARF

**Onset**

Onset is the period of time from the precipitating event to the onset of oliguria and the duration may be variable, from hours to days. The urinary output is not always decreased during this stage.

**Oliguric phase**

The speed at which this phase is established depends upon the cause of ARF. The urine output falls to <400 ml/24 h but it may remain normal or high in some cases (Redmond et al., 2004). This phase can last 3–21 days but has been known to last up to

3 months. The longer this phase then the poorer the function of the kidney becomes, with anuria being a poor prognostic indicator (Redmond et al., 2004), indicating that RRT may be required. Plasma urea increases daily by 3.6–7.1 mmol/l but this could be higher in hypercatabolic patients, and in cases of sepsis, gastrointestinal bleeding and corticosteroid use. As the GFR falls <10 ml/min, creatinine will increase by 44–133 µmol/l per day depending upon age, muscle mass or injury (Singri et al., 2003). Blood serum potassium also starts to increase to >5 mmol/l, and metabolic acidosis can occur. Once ARF is established little can be done to restore function other than to treat the patient symptomatically until function returns.

Although ARF is associated with oliguria, 30–60% of patients are not oliguric and have a urine output in excess of 500 ml/24 h. Despite this most patients in the early stages of ARF are fluid-overloaded, usually owing to a delayed recognition of ARF and exacerbated by fluid challenges in an attempt to restore urine output. Careful consideration is needed before administering fluids to a patient who has already been resuscitated as it can cause pulmonary oedema (Armitage & Tomson, 2003).

**Diuretic phase**

This phase occurs when the kidneys are beginning to recover and they start to produce large amounts of hypotonic urine (Redmond et al., 2004) and GFR starts to increase. At this stage there must be an accurate fluid balance chart to ensure that the patient does not become fluid overloaded, which may lead to pulmonary oedema. Hydration at this stage is kept to 500 ml plus the previous day's output but the dietary restrictions may be lifted according to results of urea and electrolyte tests because the kidney has now started to concentrate. Urine levels can return to normal.

**Recovery phase**

This phase is when tubular function is restored and the urea and creatinine levels start to fall. Up to 50% of patients can be left with a degree of renal damage.

## CLINICAL AND BIOCHEMICAL FEATURES ASSOCIATED WITH ARF

Clinical and biochemical features associated with ARF include:

- cardiavascular system:
  - anaemia,
  - hypertension,
  - arrhythmias;
- respiratory system:
  - pulmonary oedema causing difficulty in breathing,
  - metabolic acidosis causing Kussmauls respirations;
- neurological system:
  - altered mental state due to high urea;
- urinary system:
  - urine volume variable,
  - concentration variable depending upon cause;
- blood chemistry:
  - increase in potassium,
  - increase in urea,
  - increase in creatinine.

## INVESTIGATIONS

Diagnosis is usually by careful history-taking, a thorough physical examination and interpretation of laboratory data, ultrasound and other radiological investigations (Singri et al., 2003). Initial investigations are aimed at life-threatening features (Fry & Farrington, 2006). Specific investigations for ARF are detailed in Table 7.2.

## TREATMENT OF ARF

Protocols for the rapid and effective treatment of ARF by appropriately trained healthcare professionals should be agreed and available locally. The specific treatment of a patient who presents with ARF will now be described. The management of problems associated with ARF and RRT are discussed later in the chapter.

**Table 7.2** Investigations for ARF

| Test | Abnormality | Cause |
|---|---|---|
| **Urinalysis** | | |
| Dipstick urinalysis | Haematuria | Renal inflammatory process e.g. rapidly progressive glomerulonephritis (RPGN), rhabdomyolosis (Short & Cumming, 1999; Stevens et al., 2001; Armitage & Tomson, 2003) |
| | Proteinuria: positive protein values of 3+ or 4+ on reagent strip testing | Intrinsic renal disease, rhabdomyolosis (Stevens et al., 2001) |
| Microscopy | Red cell casts | Glomerulonephritis (Hilton, 2006) |
| | White cell casts | Interstitial nephritis, acute pyelonephritis. (Stevens et al., 2001) |
| Osmolarity | >400 mOsm/kg | Indicates pre-renal failure (Redmond et al., 2004) |
| Specific gravity | >1.010 | Pre-acute renal failure |
| | <1.012 | Acute tubular necrosis |
| Urinary sodium and electrolytes | Low urinary sodium excretion | Pre-acute renal failure |
| | High urinary sodium and low osmolarity | Rhabdomyoloysis |
| | | Acute tubular necrosis, diuretic therapy, contrast nephropathy (Redmond et al., 2004) |
| Bence Jones | Proteinuria | Myeloma (Hilton, 2006) |
| **Blood tests** | | |
| Urea and electrolytes | Increases in urea, creatinine and potassium; reduced sodium | All causes of acute renal failure (Redmond et al., 2004) |
| | Decreased calcium: there is not a significant increase until there is a 50% reduction in renal function (Mahon & Hattersley, 2002) | |

| | | |
|---|---|---|
| Full blood count and coagulation studies | Raised white cell count, platelet consumption and red cell damage | Common in ARF (Sinert & Peacock, 2006) |
| Blood cultures | Should be undertaken if infection is suspected (Fry & Farrington, 2006) | Disseminated intravascular coagulation associated with sepsis (Hilton, 2006)<br>Sepsis induced ARF, acute interstitial nephritis and haemolytic uraemic syndrome |

**Radiological investigations**

| | | |
|---|---|---|
| Renal ultrasonography | Renal size, symmetry and any evidence of obstruction | Intrarenal or post renal obstruction (Stevens et al., 2001; Armitage & Tomson, 2003; Redmond et al., 2004) |
| Renal biopsy | Abnormalities of renal tissue. Considered in all pts with normal sized non obstructed kidneys (Armitage & Tomson, 2003) | Glomerulonephritis, vasculitis (Redmond et al., 2004) |

**Virology**

| | | |
|---|---|---|
| Hepatitis B and C | | Important implications for infection control within dialysis area (Hilton, 2006) |
| HIV | | |

**Other**

| | | |
|---|---|---|
| Renal Doppler flows | | Renovascular disease (Singri et al., 2003) |
| Chest X-ray | Pulmonary oedema | Fluid overload (Redmond et al., 2004) |
| ECG | Abnormal cardiac arrhythmias | High potassium |

- Assess the patient following the ABCDE approach described in Chapter 1. Evaluate MEWS score, alert medics/outreach if necessary (see p. 298).
- Ensure that the patient has a clear airway: if the patient has altered conscious level, the airway is at risk.
- Administer high-flow oxygen using a non-rebreathe mask (Figure 1.4). Establish oxygen-saturation monitoring using a pulse oximeter.
- Insert a wide-bore intravenous (IV) cannula (e.g. 14 gauge).
- Commence IV fluids, as prescribed.
- Establish continuous ECG monitoring: electrolyte abnormalities, particularly hyperkalaemia, can cause life-threatening cardiac arrhythmias (Resuscitation Council UK, 2006).
- Insert a urinary catheter and monitor urine output closely.
- Closely monitor the patient's vital signs, fluid balance, blood glucose, blood ketones, arterial blood gases, and urea and electrolytes.
- Involve the renal physician as soon as possible.
- If the patient is confused, ensure that the environment is safe and hazard-free.
- Ensure appropriate management of specific problems associated with ARF and consider RRT (see below).

## MANAGEMENT OF SPECIFIC PROBLEMS ASSOCIATED WITH ARF

### Hypovolaemia

Hypovolaemia potentiates and exacerbates all forms of ARF. Reversal of hypovolaemia by rapid fluid infusion is often sufficient to treat ARF, but this can result in a life-threatening overload. Accurate determination of the patient's fluid status is essential (Sinert & Peacock, 2006). Regular assessment and monitoring of the patient's circulating volume should be made by:

- central venous pressure (CVP),
- strict fluid balance charts of input/output.

Strict fluid balance charts of input and output must be recorded (Armitage & Tomson, 2003). The importance of their accuracy can not be over-emphasised in order to determine fluid status of the patient.

### Fluid overload

Early signs of fluid overload are oedema of the feet, legs and sacral area, meaning that observation for any changes in skin care is important at this stage. Pulmonary oedema as a complication – normally as a result of excessive fluid resuscitation – carries a high mortality rate (Fry & Farrington, 2006). If there is significant ventilatory failure this must be dealt with first. It may be anticipated in most patients, especially those who have cardiac dysfunction and the elderly, who are volume overloaded at the outset. Observe for:

- raised respiratory rate,
- shortness of breath,
- orthopnoea.

Pharmacological treatment to offload a decompensated heart can be used (Fry & Farrington, 2006):

- IV opioids: diamorphine 2.5–5 mg but it needs to be used with caution in patients with respiratory failure;
- IV infusion of glyceryl trinitrate 50 mg/ml in 0.9% sodium chloride at a rate of 2–20 ml/h, keeping systolic blood pressure >95 mmHg.

To provoke a diuresis use Frusemide 250 mg in 50 ml of 0.9% sodium chloride in 1 hr. An effect is normally seen in 1–2 hrs (Fry & Farrington, 2006).

The theoretical rationale for the use of loop diuretics in ARF is the inhibition of the sodium/potassium/chloride pump in the thick ascending limb of the loop of Henle. This leads to a subsequent decrease in sodium, potassium and ATPase activity. This should reduce the oxygen requirements of the cells and the susceptibility to ischaemic damage, but there are scarce data to support this.

A meta-analysis undertaken by Ho and Sheridan (2006) found that furesomide is ineffective in the prevention and treatment of ARF because it does not:

- reduce in-hospital mortality,
- significantly reduce the need for RRT,
- influence the number of dialysis sessions required until recovery of renal function.

If the interventions are not successful fluid removal is by RRT in the form of continuous renal replacement therapy (CRRT), also known as haemofiltration, intermittent haemodialysis (IHD) or peritoneal dialysis. The choice of treatment is determined by the patient's needs, location of the treatment and cardio/respiratory support.

To avoid fluid overload a maintenance regime should be started which takes into account renal and insensible losses. The aim is a positive balance of 500 ml per day + 25 ml.

### Cardiovascular instability

Cardiovascular instability is the most common complication of extra-corporeal RRT (Thomas & Harris, 2002) because of:

- instability in most critically ill patients,
- failure of compensatory mechanisms.

As a result many patients cannot tolerate the wide swings in hydration status and high rates of ultrafiltration as in IHD, so CRRT is deemed to be less vigorous as fluid can be removed slowly. CRRT is also characterised by compensatory vasoconstriction which improves vascular stability, whereas clearance of vasoconstrictors by IHD may exacerbate hypotension (Thomas & Harris, 2002). CRRT removes sodium and water without causing haemodynamic instability.

### Dopamine

Low-dose dopamine has previously been advocated by intensive care units to protect renal function; this alleged benefit is now in dispute (Debaveye & Van der Berghe, 2004). Dopamine reduces splanchic perfusion, depresses respiration and suppresses the release and function of the anterior pituitary hormone. Dopamine worsens renal function in both hypovolaemic or normovolaemic patients. At present its routine use in ARF is not justified (Pierce et al., 2002).

### Hyperkalaemia

This is the most common and potentially dangerous complication of ARF. A reduction in the GFR leads to a reduction in renal potassium excretion, leading to hyperkalaemia which can also be potentiated by:

- NSAIDs,
- ACEIs,
- ARBs,
- potassium-sparing diuretics,
- trimethoprin.

Release of potassium into extracellular fluid can cause necrosis, rhabdomyolysis and haemolysis. Potassium-excreted hydrogen ions enter the cells and uraemic acidosis occurs. ECG changes can occur (Table 7.3).

Treatment for hyperkalaemia is described below.

- Stabilisation of the myocardium produces a more normal ECG without affecting serum potassium if P wave or QRS changes are present: administer a bolus of 10–20 ml of 10% calcium gluconate in 100 ml of 5% dextrose over 2–5 min. Calcium gluconate is preferred over calcium chloride because of the high

**Table 7.3** ECG changes associated with hyperkalaemia

| | |
|---|---|
| Peaked and tented T waves | Potassium >6.5 mmol/l |
| Flattening of P wave and prolongation of QRS complex | Potassium >7.0 mmol/l |
| Sine waves | Potassium 8.0–9.0 mmol/l |
| Ventricular fibrillation or asystole | Potassium >9.0 mmol/l |

risk of tissue damage if extravasation occurs. Calcium gluconate can potentiate the cardiac toxicity of digoxin so all patients who are taking this drug should be given the same dosage but over 30 min (Fry & Farrington, 2006).

- To reduce serum potassium concentration: fast-acting soluble insulin 10 units IV in 50 ml of 50% dextrose over 10–20 min; a reduction in potassium occurs in <10 min (Singri et al., 2003; Fry & Farrington, 2006). Dextrose (50%) is also administered to counteract the insulin, preventing hypoglycaemia from occurring. Blood glucose should be monitored for 6 h as up to 75% of patients can develop hypoglycaemia (Fry & Farrington, 2006).

Or

- calcium resonium or resonium A 15 g three times a day.

Or

- RRT: haemodialysis.

### Metabolic acidosis

Severe metabolic acidosis (blood pH <7.2) usually accompanies ARF (Fry & Farrington, 2006). A blood pH of <7.2 can be due to renal dysfunction or an underlying illness. In ARF there is increased acid production from tissue hypoxia and protein catabolism, and the kidneys fail to regenerate bicarbonate ions and excrete hydrogen ions into the urine. This leads to an acid/base imbalance.

To reverse acidosis sodium bicarbonate 8.4% can be administered intravenously, although complications can occur:

- worsening intracellular acidosis but improved blood pH; this is known as paradoxical acidosis,
- overshoot metabolic acidosis,
- hypernatraemia,
- extravasation injury.

Sodium bicarbonate can be used in IHD as this provides better control over serum bicarbonate levels. Lactate is normally used as a replacement fluid in CRRT. Lactate has to be converted into bicarbonate by the liver. This may be compromised in acutely ill patients, which can result in hyperlactacidaemia, resulting in myocardial depression (Bihl, 2001). Therefore lactate free solutions are frequently used.

## Uraemic pericarditis

As the urea rises to >35 mmol/l then the risk of developing uraemic pericarditis becomes problematic. The patient will complain of chest pain when sitting back. The diagnosis is made using an echocardiogram and once urea levels begin to fall the pericarditis resolves.

## Haemorrhage

Critically ill patients with ARF frequently have anti-coagulation and bleeding abnormalities (Bihl, 2001). This can occur as a result of decreased platelet function due to uraemic syndrome and the use of anti-coagulants in RRT. Anti-coagulation is necessary for efficient haemostasis and to stop clotting in the extracorporeal circuit in RRT.

Heparin is the commonest anti-coagulation method for patients with no bleeding and a normal anti-coagulation profile. The aim of therapy is to anticoagulate the extracorporeal circuit, not the patient, thereby avoiding complications and extending circuit life (Dirkes, 2000); if heparin is used for a prolonged time it may cause thrombotic thrombocytopenia (Thomas & Harris, 2000). Regular flushing with 0.9% sodium chloride without anticoagulants is an alternative method but it is labour-intensive. Amanzaden and Reilly (2006) suggest using other methods of anti-coagulation: regional (in the circuit) heparin and protamine, regional citrate, nafamostst, platelet inhibiting agents, e.g., prostacyclin and thrombin antagonists, e.g., recombinant hirudin. Low molecular weight heparins and heparinoids have also been utilised. The absence of anti-coagulation increases the downtime of CRRT, resulting in less-effective treatments and increased cost of care (Amanzaden & Reilly, 2006). Coagulopathies may need to be corrected with blood products and vitamin K (Fry & Farrington, 2006).

**Nutrition**

In hypercatabolic ARF patients become nutritionally deficient in protein and energy requirements. Catabolism is when energy requirements exceed the supply of available carbohydrates resulting in the breakdown of body fats and protein stores. Forty per cent of patients with ARF are malnourished (Fiaccadori et al., 1999). The primary goals of nutrition in ARF are:

- maintaining or improving nutritional status by providing adequate calories and nutrients without exacerbating metabolic derangements,
- enhancement of wound healing,
- supporting immune function (Strejic, 2005).

CRRT allows room for hyperalimination (Thomas & Harris, 2002).

Alterations in protein or amino acids, carbohydrates and lipid metabolism as well as fluid, electrolyte and acid/base balance need to be considered when providing nutritional therapy in patients with ARF. Calorie needs of patients remains controversial and appear to be based on the degree of dysfunction and the need for RRT (Strejic, 2005). RRT may also clear some vitamins and minerals so supplemented vitamins are needed.

A fall in protein catabolism and oxygen consumption also causes a reduction in body temperature (Jones, 2004), which in some cases may be beneficial as compensatory vasoconstriction may cause cardiovascular stability (Thomas & Harris, 2002). Nutritional replacement can be given by enteral or parental methods (Strejic, 2005).

*Enteral nutritional replacement*

Although a patient with ARF may experience an increased incidence of gastrointestinal problems the gastrointestinal tract should be utilised to maintain gut integrity. The benefits of enteral feeding are:

- volume control,
- use of more concentrated speciality formulas,
- cost effectiveness.

*Parenteral nutritional replacement*
Parenteral nutrition may be necessary in gastrointestinal dysmotility. Electrolytes may be added as necessary; the tolerance of higher dextrose solutions and lipid emulsions may be poorer in ARF.

## Solute clearance during RRT
There are increased morbidity outcomes in patients who have better solute clearances. Although IHD can clear toxins, problems can occur because they accumulate rapidly in the interdialytic period. Rapid removal may lead to disequilibrium variably manifested by:

- cerebral oedema,
- cardiac arrhythmias,
- decreased splanchic perfusion.

CRRT avoids these problems but the following problems can still result:

- electrolyte disturbance due to fluid substitution,
- increased fluid removal leading to a negative sodium balance (= hyponatraemia),
- magnesium, phosphate and calcium depletion especially when a citrate is used as an anti-coagulant.

## Removal of inflammatory mediators
Accumulation of toxic middle molecules are thought to contribute to organ dysfunction and cardiovascular instability in critically ill and septic patients (Thomas & Harris, 2002).

## Biocompatibility and membrane interactions
Exposure of blood to bio-incompatible surfaces may cause a low-grade inflammatory response (Dirkes, 2000). There is no evidence to suggest any difference between biocompatible and bio-incompatible membranes in treating patients with ARF; biocompatible membranes should be used because they inhibit the activity of inflammatory mediators.

**Table 7.4** Sources of infection

| Infection | Cause | Prevention and treatment |
|---|---|---|
| Septicaemia | Cannulation | Aseptic technique |
| | Venous or arterial catheterisation | Observation |
| Pneumonia | Pulmonary oedema | Strict fluid balance |
| | Hypostasis | Prevent fluid overload |
| | Bedrest | Chest physiotherapy |
| Urinary tract | Urethral catheters | Remove catheter if oliguric |
| infection | Low urine output | |

### Control of infection

Infection may be a causative factor or a complication. Uraemia causes a reduction in the efficiency of the patient's immune system (Redmond et al., 2004). The patient may not always have a pyrexia because of anaemia and therefore the patient may have a sub-acute infection. The sources of infection are shown in Table 7.4.

### Mobility

If undergoing CRRT it is difficult to move patients to different departments for investigations, as CRRT needs to be discontinued which reduces patients treatment times (Dirkes, 2000).

### Renal replacement therapy (RRT)

There is limited evidence to guide decisions on when to commence RRT (Armitage and Tomson, 2003; Palevsky, 2006); however, the need to commence RRT can be based on several factors:

- the degree of hypercatabolism;
- patient's size;
- clinical assessment of volume status and metabolic control (Bihl, 2001);
- urea >30–50 mmol/l;
- plasma creatinine >500 µmol/l;
- hyperkalaemia unresponsive to medical therapy (Fry & Farrington, 2006);
- severity of metabolic acidosis;

- pulmonary oedema;
- drug overdose with dialysable toxin;
- symptoms of uraemia:
  - nausea/vomiting,
  - severe itching,
  - fits,
  - pericarditis,
  - bleeding.

A number of strategies can be employed in the treatment of ARF (Armitage & Tomson, 2003; Rabindranath et al., 2006):

- continuous RRT (haemofiltration):
  - slow continuous ultrafiltration (SCUF),
  - continuous arteriovenous haemofiltration (CAVH),
  - continuous venovenous haemofiltration (CVVH),
  - continuous venovenous diafiltration (CWHDF);
- IHD,
- peritoneal dialysis,
- slow extended daily dialysis (SLEDD).

Despite growing utilisation of CRRT (Riegal, 2003) over IHD superiority of CRRT is not demonstrated (Palevsky, 2006). CRRT is recommended for patients with multi-organ failure and cardiac instability and IHD for patients with single-organ failure who are stable.

### Continuous RRT (haemofiltration)
Haemofiltration is a 24-hours-a-day, 7-days-a-week process which removes fluids and solutes slowly, correcting electrolyte and metabolic disturbances associated with ARF (Paton, 2003). This process is continued until renal function is restored or the patient can tolerate haemodialysis.

#### Slow continuous ultrafiltration (SCUF)
SCUF requires placement of both arterial and venous catheters and utilises the patient's mean arterial pressure to drive blood

through the circuit. Solute clearance is by ultrafiltration and replacement fluid is not used. It is useful for volume overload but not solute clearance.

### Continuous arteriovenous haemofiltration (CAVH)

CAVH is achieved by blood passing from an arterial catheter and returning via a venous catheter. It is dependent on the patient's blood pressure (Paton, 2003). This form of CRRT is rarely used today and is not recommended (Bihl, 2001).

### Continuous venovenous haemofiltration (CVVH)

This is the preferred method with ease of access and reduced arterial complications. The problems of relying upon the patient's blood pressure to force the blood through circuit are overcome by adding a blood pump to guarantee blood flow through the haemofilter. This in turn increases the ultrafiltration rate. A double-lumen catheter is inserted into the jugular, femoral or subclavian veins to provide vascular access. Blood flows from the access into the extracorporeal circuit and into the haemofilter. The haemofilter has multiple semi-permeable hollow fibres that fill with blood. Small- to medium-sized solutes pass through the haemofilter by convection and ultrafiltration takes place; the fluid collected in the drainage bag is called ultrafiltrate. Ultrafiltration rates are 35 ml/ kg per h and approximately up to 2 litres are removed hourly. Replacement fluid is used to replace ultrafiltration. Solute and fluid are removed slowly for 24 h every day but normally for 24–72 h at a time. The following solutes are removed:

- sodium,
- potassium,
- phosphate,
- ionised calcium,
- urea,
- creatinine,
- glucose,
- drugs not bound to protein.

*Continuous venovenous haemodiafiltration (CWHDF)*

This is similar to CVVH. Thomas and Harris (2000) provide solute and fluid removal by both diffusion (IHD) and convection (CRRT) simultaneously. This modality is the one most frequently used in the critically ill patient.

*Slow extended daily dialysis (SLEDD)*

SLEDD combines both CRRT and IHD. The treatment lasts for 6–12 h, using blood flows of 100–150 ml/min with dialysate flows of 100–300 ml/min. Variations in flow rates and length of dialysis are based on individual needs. The shorter the treatment time the less anti-coagulant will be used.

## Intermitent haemodialysis (IHD)

IHD is an extracorporeal process of removing soluble substances and water from the blood across a semi-permeable membrane by diffusion and filtration and the use of transmembrane pressure. IHD requires dual venous access and is carried out for a period of 3–5 h, three to seven times a week. Solute removal is by diffusion and is rapid and efficient (Murray & Hall, 2000). It is a complicated procedure in hypotensive patients, fluid removal is less than haemofiltration, usually 500–2000 ml because of the risk of hypotension and further renal damage (Manns et al., 1997).

Short sessions are provided initially; the length of time is then built up gradually either daily or on alternate days. It is technically a complex procedure and needs to be carried out by highly trained nurses (Lamiere et al., 1998). There is more accurate control of fluid removal than with CAVH.

## Peritoneal dialysis

Peritoneal dialysis removes solutes and water from the body across the peritoneal membrane through diffusion, filtration and osmosis. A dialysate solution is administered via a temporary catheter into the peritoneal cavity, where it stays for a prescribed period of time and is then drained (Dirkes, 2000). The use of peritoneal dialysis is contraindicated in:

- recent abdominal surgery,
- respiratory failure,
- peritonitis.

Rarely used in the treatment of ARF in developed countries, peritoneal dialysis may have a role where vascular access or anti-coagulation are not available or when gentle fluid removal is required or the resources for blood-based approaches are not available. The outcomes are poor because of the high risk of infection. It does not require large doses of anti-coagulation and is tolerated well by acutely ill patients, but ventilated patients may experience respiratory pressures due to fluid pressing on the diaphragm.

Treatment is by using 1500–2000 ml over short periods of time (60–90 min) or by using a peritoneal dialysis cycler and building up in increasing doses to 2000 ml. Two litres of 4.25% dextrose with two exchanges per hour can remove 500–700 ml/h in fluid-overloaded patients. Short peritoneal dialysis cycles can cause hypokalaemia so potassium may need to be added to the bags. Hypercatabolic ARF peritoneal dialysis cannot maintain optimal uraemic or pH control, which is partly explained by the peritoneum being poorly perfused. Some of the complications are peritonitis and leakage from the access site.

## SURVIVAL AND RECOVERY OF RENAL FUNCTION

Thomas and Harris (2000) identified through a meta-analysis that there is a 15% reduction in mortality with CRRT compared with IHD, although CRRT is not suitable for all groups of patients (Table 7.5). Although the meta-analysis by Kellum et al. (2002) did not identify any significant differences in survival rate when comparing CRRT with IHD, Rabindranath et al. (2006) identified flaws in the meta-analysis and suggest that it should be repeated using Cochrane review methodology.

CVVHD as compared with IHD does not reduce mortality nor does it influence the length of stay, haemodynamic instability or recovery of renal function (Tonelli et al., 2002; Uehlinger et al., 2005).

**Table 7.5** Advantages and disadvantages of CRRT and IHD

|  | CRRT | IHD |
| --- | --- | --- |
| Advantages | Increased haemodynamic stability | Reduced systemic bleeding |
|  | Improved fluid control | Increased time for diagnostic investigations |
|  | More effective control of acid/base balance and electrolyte balance | Better control of hyperkalaemia |
|  | Improved removal of toxins | More cost effective |
|  | Removal of inflammatory mediators | Shorter stay in intensive care |
|  | Improved pulmonary gas exchange |  |
|  | Improved nutritional support |  |
| Disadvantages | Increased risk of systemic bleeding | Difficult haemodynamic control |
|  | Increased risk of problems with vascular access | Availability of dialysis staff |
|  | Higher risk of filter and extra-corporeal circuit clotting | Inadequate dialysis dose |
|  | Less mobilisation of patient | Inadequate fluid control |
|  | Increased cost/resources/staff | Not suitable for patients with intercranial hypertension |
|  |  | Does not remove cytokines |

Sources: adapted from Fry and Farrington (2006) and Rabindranath et al. (2006).

## CONCLUSION

ARF is a common medical emergency with significant mortality. It is characterised by a sudden decline in renal function over hours or days. It can occur in people with previously normal kidney function or underlying kidney disease (Department of Health, 2005) and often requires emergency treatment in the form of RRT. Prompt recognition and effective treatment of ARF is paramount if the risk of complications is to be minimised.

## REFERENCES

Amanzaden, J & Reilly, RF (2006) Anticoagulation and continuous replacement therapy. *Seminars in Dialysis* **19**(4), 311–16

Armitage, AJ & Tomson, C (2003) Acute renal failure. *Medicine* **31**(6), 43–8

Armstrong, T & Bircher, G (2002) Acute renal failure. In Thomas, N (ed.), *Renal Nursing*, 2nd edn, pp. 103–24. Elsevier, London

Bellomo, R, Ronco, C, Kellum, JA & the Acute Dialysis Quality Initiative Workgroup (2004) Acute renal failure definition, outcome measures, animal models, fluid therapy and information technology needs. Second International Consensus Conference ADQI Group. *Critical Care* 8, 204–212

Bennett-Jones, DN (2006) Early intervention in acute renal failure. *British Medical Journal* **333**, 406–7

Bihl, G (2001) Non-dialytic management of acute renal failure in the ICU. *British Journal of Renal Medicine* **6**(2), 6–8

Block, CA & Schoolwerth, AC (2006) The epidemiology and outcome of acute renal failure and the impact on chronic kidney disease. *Seminars in Dialysis* **19**(6), 450–4

Chen Y-C, Chen C-Y, Hsu H-H, Yang, C-W & Fang, J-T (2002) Apache III scoring system in critically ill patients with acute renal failure requiring dialysis. *Dialysis and Transplantation* **31**(4), 222–9, 233

Debaveye, Y & Van der Berghe, GH (2004) Is there still a place for dopamine in the modern intensive care unit. *Anaesthesia & Analgesia* **98**, 461–8

Department of Health (2005) *The National Service Framework for Renal Services. Part 2: Chronic Kidney Disease, Acute Renal Failure and End of Life Care*. Department of Health, London

Dirkes, SM (2000) Continuous renal replacement therapy: dialytic therapy for acute renal failure in intensive care. *Nephrology Nursing Journal* **27**(6), 581–93

Esson, ML & Schrier, R (2002) Diagnosis and treatment of acute tubular necrosis. *Annals of Internal Medicine* **137**(9), 744–52

Feest, TG, Round, A & Hamad, S (1993) Incidence of severe acute renal failure in adults: results of a community based study. *British Medical Journal* **306**(6876), 481–3

Fiaccadori, E, Lombardi, M, Leonardi, S, Rotelli, CF, Tortorella, G & Borghetti, A (1999) Prevalence and outcome associated with pre-existing nutrition in acute renal failure. *Journal of American Society of Nephrologists* **10**, 581–93

Fry, AC & Farrington, K (2006) Management of acute renal failure *Postgraduate Medical Journal* **85**, 106–16

Galley, H (2000) Can acute renal failure be prevented. *Journal of the Royal College of Surgeons of Edinburgh* **45**, 45–50

Hegarty, J, Middleton, RJ, Krebs, M, Hussain, H, Cheung, C, Ledson, T, et al. (2005) Severe acute renal failure in adults, place of care, incidence and outcomes *Quarterly Journal of Medicine* **98**(9), 661–6

Hilton, R (2006) Acute renal failure. *British Medical Journal* **333**, 786–90

Ho, KM & Sheridan, D (2006) Meta-analysis of frusemide to prevent or treat acute renal failure. *British Medical Journal* **333**, 420–3

Jones, S (2004) Heat loss and continuous renal replacement therapy. *AACN Clinical Issues* **15**(2), 223–30

Kellum, JA, Angus, D, Johnson, J, Leblanc, M, Griffin, M, Ramakrishnan, N & Linde-Zwirble, WT (2002) Continuous versus intermittent renal replacement therapy: a meta-analysis. *Intensive Care Medicine* **28**(1), 29–37

Lamiere, N, Van Biesen, W, Vanholder, R & Colardjin, F (1998) The place of intermittent haemodialysis in the treatment of acute renal failure in the ICU patient. *Kidney International Supplement* **66**, 110–19

Lamiere, N, Van Biesen, W & Vanholder, R (2005) Acute renal failure. *Lancet* **365**(9457), 417–30

Mahon, A & Hattersley, J (2002) Renal investigations. In Thomas, N (ed.), *Renal Nursing*, 2nd edn, pp. 143–70. Elsevier, London

Manns, M, Sigler, MH & Teehan, BP (1997) Intradialytic renal haemodynamics – potential consequences for the management of the patient with acute renal failure. *Nephrology, Dialysis and Transplantation* **12**(5), 870–2

McCulloch, P, Wolyn, R, Rocher, LL, Levin, RN & O'Neill, WW (1997) Acute renal failure after coronary intervention incidence, risk factors and relationship in mortality. *American Journal of Medicine* **103**(5), 368–74

Mehta, R & Chertow, GM (2003) Acute renal failure definitions and classifications: time for a change. *Journal American Society of Nephrology* **14**, 2178–87

Metcalfe, W, Simpson, M, Khan, IH, Prescott, GJ, Simpson, K, Smith, WCS & MacLeod, AM (2002) Acute renal failure requiring renal replacement therapy: incidence and outcome. *Quarterly Journal of Medicine* **95**, 579–83

Murray, P & Hall, J (2000) Renal replacement therapy for acute renal failure. *American Journal of Respiratory and Critical Care Medicine* **162**(3), 777–81

Paganini, E, Halstenberg, W & Goormastic, M (1996) Acute renal failure requiring dialysis. The introduction of a new module. *Clinical Nephrology* **46**, 206–11

Palevsky, PM (2006) Dialysis modality and dosing strategy in acute renal failure. *Seminars in Dialysis* **19**(2), 165–72

Paton, M (2003) Continuous renal replacement therapy. Slow but steady. *Nursing* **33**(6), 48–50

Pierce, J, Morris, D & Clancy, R (2002) Understanding renal dose dopamine. *Journal of Infusion Nursing* **25**(6), 365–71

Rabindranath, KS, Muirhead, N & Macleod, AM (2006) Intermittent versus continuous renal replacement therapy for acute renal failure in adults. *Cochrane Database of Systematic Reviews* **2**, CD003773

Redmond, A, McDevitt, M & Barnes, S (2004) Acute renal failure: recognition and treatment in ward patients. *Nursing Standard* **18**(22), 46–55

Riegal, W (2003) Continuous renal replacement therapy in acute renal failure. *Kidney and Blood Pressure Research* **26**(2), 123–7

Resuscitation Council UK (2006) *Advanced Life Support Provider Manual*, 5th edn. Resuscitation Council UK, London

Robertson, S, Newbigging, CG, Isles, A, Bramman, A, Allan, A & Norrie, J (2002) High incidence of renal failure requiring short term dialysis: a prospective observational study. *Quarterly Journal of Medicine* **95**, 585–90

Royal College of Physicians and Renal Association (2007) *The Changing Face of Renal Medicine in the UK. The Future of the Speciality.* Report of a Working Party. Royal College of Physicians, London

Short, A & Cumming, A (1999) ABC of intensive care: renal support. *British Medical Journal* **319**(7201), 41–4

Sinert, R & Peacock, PR (2006) Renal failure: acute. www.medscape.com/files/emedicine/topic500.htm (accessed 21 January 2008)

Singri, N, Ahya, S, Shubhada, N & Levin, ML (2003) Acute renal failure. *Journal of the American Medical Association* **289**(6), 747–51

Stevens, PE, Tamimi, NA, Al-Hasani, MK, Mikhail, AI, Kearney, E, Lapworth, R, et al. (2001) Non specialist management of acute renal failure. *Quarterly Journal of Medicine* **94**(10), 533–40

Strejic, JM (2005) Considerations in the nutritional management of patients with acute renal failure. *Haemodialysis International* **9**(2), 135–42

Thomas, C & Harris, CH (2002) Problems and advantages of continuous renal replacement therapy. *Nephrology* **7**, 110–14

Tonelli, M, Manns, B & Feller-Kopman, D (2002) Acute renal failure in the intensive care unit: a systematic review of the impact of dialytic modality on mortality and renal recovery. *American Journal of Kidney Diseases* **40**(5), 875–85

Uehlinger, DE, Jakob, S, Ferrari, P, Eichelberger, M, Huynh-Do, U, Marti, P, et al. (2005) Comparison of continuous and intermittent renal replacement therapy. *Nephrology, Dialysis and Transplantation* **20**(8), 1630–7

# 8 | Gastrointestinal Emergencies

## Beverley Ewens

## INTRODUCTION

Gastrointestinal emergencies can be life-threatening. Regardless of the underlying cause, the initial priorities centre on the ABCDE approach and ensuring that a high concentration of oxygen is administered at an early stage. Intravenous access will need to be secured and fluid resuscitation may need to be commenced. Ensuring that the patient is kept nil by mouth until told otherwise is sensible and the early involvement of senior medical help is paramount.

The aim of this chapter is to help the reader understand the management of gastrointestinal emergencies.

## LEARNING OUTCOMES

At the end of this chapter the reader will be able to discuss treatment for:

❏ acute liver failure.
❏ acute pancreatitis,
❏ gastrointestinal haemorrhage,

## ACUTE LIVER FAILURE (ALF)

Liver disease is a major cause of morbidity and mortality in the critical care setting with overall mortality estimated at 90–97% without liver transplantation (Marrero et al., 2003). ALF or fulminant hepatic failure (FHF) is a consequence of severe liver injury in the absence of pre-existing liver disease and is a potentially reversible condition (McGuiness, 2007). Progressive hepatocyte necrosis results in the dysfunction of virtually every major organ system (Kulkarni & Cronin, 2005). Liver cells become injured and die and are replaced by scar tissue. ALF is defined as the onset of encephalopathy within 8 weeks of the onset of liver-related symptoms (Kulkarni & Cronin, 2005).

## Pathogenesis

A consequence of ALF is cerebral oedema and this is associated with a mortality rate of 30–50% (McGuiness, 2007). Elevated levels of ammonia are thought to be involved in its development (Sood & Jones, 2006). A dysfunction of cerebral blood flow autoregulation, cerebral vasodilation and a disrupted blood–brain barrier all contribute to fluid loss into the interstitial space and the development of raised intracranial pressure (ICP) (Kulkarni & Cronin, 2005). Another consequence of ALF is multi-organ dysfunction syndrome (MODS), which often is observed in the context of a hyperdynamic circulatory state that mimics sepsis (low systemic vascular resistance); therefore, circulatory insufficiency and poor organ perfusion possibly either initiate or promote complications of ALF (Sood & Jones, 2006). Elevated serum concentrations of bacterial endotoxin, tumour necrosis factor-alpha, interleukin-1 and interleukin-6 have been found in ALF, but the specific roles of these inflammatory mediators are unclear.

## Causes

The causes of ALF are varied and include the following.
Infective:

- hepatitis A and B (rarely hepatitis C),
- Epstein–Barr virus,
- cytomegalovirus,
- echovirus,
- varicella (chicken pox),
- salmonella,

- tuberculosis,
- sepsis,
- malaria,
- leptospirosis.

Drugs:

- acetaminophen (paracetamol) (39%),
- allopurinol,
- amioderone,
- antibiotics,
- carbamazepine,
- halothane,
- ecstacy,
- isoniazid,
- non-steriodal anti-inflammatory drugs (NSAIDs),
- phenytoin,
- sodium valporate.

Toxins:

- mushroom poisons (e.g. *Amanita* mushroom),
- herbal medicines,
- carbon tetrachloride,
- yellow phosphorous,
- industrial solvents.

Metabolic:

- galactosaemia (deficiency of an enzyme catalysing the conversion of galactose to glucose),
- tyrosinaemia (disorder of tyrosine metabolism),
- hereditary fructose intolerance,
- Wilson's disease,
- neonatal haemochromatosis,
- Niemann–Pick disease,
- mitochondrial cytopathies,
- congenital disorders of glycosylation.

Vascular:

- Budd–Chiari syndrome,
- shock,
- heat stroke,
- acute cardiac failure,
- cardiomyopathies.

Infiltrative:

- leukaemia,
- lymphoma,
- acute fatty liver of pregnancy.

(Source: Day & Taylor, 2006)

## Clinical features

- jaundice: not always present;
- right upper quadrant tenderness: not always present;
- hepatomegaly: characteristically seen in viral hepatitis or Budd–Chiari syndrome, but may be seen in congestive heart failure;
- cerebral oedema: with resultant increased ICP, including papilloedema, hypertension and bradycardia;
- ascites: develops rapidly, particularly in Budd–Chiari syndrome;
- hematemesis or melena: due to upper gastrointestinal bleeding;
- hypotension and tachycardia: due to reduced systemic vascular resistance.

(Source: Sood & Jones, 2006)

## Diagnosis

Diagnosis requires careful history-taking to ascertain toxin exposure and pre-existing liver disease, clinical examination and biochemical analysis. Diagnosis is made upon evidence of:

- coagulopathy,
- rapid deterioration of liver function,
- altered mental state: indicative of encephalopathy (Table 8.1).

**Table 8.1** West Haven classification of hepatic encephalopathy

| | |
|---|---|
| Stage 0 | Minimal hepatic encephalopathy. Lack of detectable changes in personality or behaviour. Minimal changes in memory, concentration, intellectual function and co-ordination. Asterixis (involuntary hand movements) absent. |
| Stage 1 | Trivial lack of awareness. Shortened attention span. Impaired addition or subtraction. Hypersomnia, insomnia or inversion of sleep pattern. Euphoria, depression or irritability. Mild confusion. Slowing of ability to perform mental tasks. Asterixis can be detected. |
| Stage 2 | Lethargy or apathy. Disorientation. Inappropriate behaviour. Slurred speech. Obvious asterixis. Drowsiness, gross defecits in ability to perform mental tasks, obvious personality changes, inappropriate behaviour and intermittent disorientation usually regarding time. |
| Stage 3 | Somnolent but rousable, unable to perform mental tasks, disorientation about time and place, marked confusion, amnesia, occasional fits of rage, present but incomprehensible speech. |
| Stage 4 | Coma with or without response to painful stimuli. |

Source: Wolf (2007).

## Investigations

Investigations that should be undertaken to ascertain the severity and cause of ALF and any existing organ dysfunction include:

- serum glucose: may be very low due to impaired gluconeogenesis;
- urea and electrolytes;
- full blood count: may indicate thrombocytopenia;
- liver function tests:
  - serum bilirubin: (increases as hepatic function deteriorates) albumin, bilirubin, alkaline phosphatase, aspartate aminotransferase, alanine aminotransferase,
  - levels of the transaminases (aspartate aminotransferase, serum glutamic oxaloacetic transaminase, alanine aminotransferase): often dramatically elevated due to hepatocellular necrosis;
- serum ammonia: may be dramatically elevated;
- serum lactate: elevated level may reflect reduced tissue perfusion;
- arterial blood gases: may indicate hypoxaemia;

- serum creatinine: may be elevated, signifying the development of hepatorenal syndrome;
- blood cultures: risk of infection is increased with ALF;
- international normalised ratio: will indicate coagulopathy if raised;
- serological assays for hepatitis A and B;
- acetaminophen levels;
- toxin levels;
- upper right quadrant abdominal ultrasound: unless cause of ALF has been ascertained;
- CT abdomen: particularly if transplant is planned.

(Source: Sood & Jones, 2006)

**Treatment**

The management of the symptoms of ALF is initially supportive.

- Assess the patient following the ABCDE approach described in Chapter 1. Evaluate MEWS score, alert medics/outreach if necessary (see p. 298).
- Ensure that the patient has a clear airway; consider airway adjuncts.
- Administer high-flow oxygen using a non-rebreathe mask.
- Progress to invasive ventilation when encephalopathy is grade 3 or more.
- Establish oxygen-saturation monitoring using a pulse oximeter. Closely monitor the patient's breathing.
- Initiate regular recordings of vital signs and neurological state, such as the Glasgow Coma Scale (GCS).
- Insert a wide-bore intravenous (IV) cannula or preferably a central venous catheter (CVC; e.g. 14 gauge).
- Monitor ICP with intraventricular catheter (in specialised units only): aim for <20 mmHg (insert when the international normalised ratio (INR) has been normalised). Administer mannitol for osmotic diuresis therapy for persistent intracranial hypertension.

- Aim for a cerebral perfusion pressure (CPP) of >60 mmHg (CPP = mean arterial pressure − ICP); utilise inotropes as necessary to maintain mean arterial pressure.
- Position the patient at 30°, head up, which allows optimal jugular drainage.
- Ensure nose and sternal alignment to enhance venous drainage through the jugular vein and reduce ICP by reducing blood in the cranial vault.
- Monitor blood sugar levels: the condition can require aggressive administration of 10% dextrose centrally.
- Correct electrolyte abnormalities with IV supplements.
- Administer broad-spectrum antibiotic if infection is suspected.
- Correct coagulopathy with fresh frozen plasma.
- Administer recombinant Factor VII for coagulopathy: fresh frozen plasma can normalise the prothrombin time for up to 6 h.
- Administer IV sedation: for example, propofol which crosses the blood–brain barrier easily and reduces brain metabolic rate.
- Administer bolus IV sedation prior to interventions to minimise a transient rise in ICP.
- Actively cool the patient to 33–35°C: this reduces cerebral blood flow and ICP.
- Administer aperients to avoid straining at stool and a rise in ICP. There is no evidence to support the use of aperients to reduce ammonia levels for patients with hepatic cerebral oedema.
- Early intervention is required with continuous renal replacement therapy for renal failure.
- Initiate early enteral feeding to maintain gut integrity and the natural elimination of gut-derived toxins (O'Neal et al., 2006).
- Liver transplantation.
- Consider extracorporeal systems for acute on chronic liver failure: Molecular Adsorbent Recirculating System (MARS™)

or Fractionated Plasma Separation Adsorption and Dialysis System (Promethius™). Systems have demonstrated the removal of cytokines from plasma and may exert benefit in acute on chronic liver failure.

(Sources: Marrero et al., 2003; Day & Taylor, 2006; Stadbauer et al., 2006; McGuiness, 2007)

## Complications

The complications of acute liver failure include:

- hypoglycaemia,
- metabolic acidosis,
- acute renal failure,
- sepsis,
- acute respiratory distress syndrome,
- MODS.
- cerebral oedema,
- brain herniation and brain stem death,

(Source: Starr & Hand, 2002)

## SEVERE ACUTE PANCREATITIS

Pancreatitis is an inflammation of the pancreas which can be acute or chronic. It is a potentially life-threatening condition with an associated mortality rate of 2–15% (Hughes, 2004). Diagnosis and mortality predictions in severe acute pancreatitis are detailed in Ranson's criteria (Table 8.2).

## Causes

Causes of acute pancreatitis include:

- mechanical:
  - biliary obstruction, for example gallstones (35%),
  - abdominal trauma,
  - endoscopic procedures, for example endoscopic retrograde cholangiopancreatography (ERCP),
  - malignancy: ampullary or pancreatic tumour,
  - surgical procedures,
  - ampullary stenosis;

**Table 8.2** Ranson's criteria

| At admission | Age >55  years |
|---|---|
| | White blood cell count >16/μl |
| | Serum glucose level >11.1 mmol/l |
| | Serum lactate >350 IU/l |
| | Aspartate aminotransferase >250 IU/l |
| During initial 48 hours | Haematocrit decrease >10% |
| | Blood urea nitrogen increase >5 mg/dl (>1.8 mmol/l) |
| | Calcium <8 mg/dl (<2 mmol/l) |
| | PaO$_2$ <8 kPa (<60 mmHg) |
| | Base deficit >4 mEq/l |
| | Fluid replacement >6 litres |

For a diagnosis of severe acute pancreatitis three or more of the above criteria must be present.

Mortality rates: 0–2 criteria met = 1%; 3–4 criteria met = 16%; 5–6 criteria met = 40%; 7 or more criteria met = 100%.

- toxins and drugs:
  - alcohol abuse (40%),
  - corticosteroids,
  - NSAIDs,
  - frusemide,
  - tetracyclin,
  - sulfonamides,
  - opiates;
- infectious:
  - *Staphylococcus*,
  - viral; hepatitis, mumps, rubella, HIV, Epstein–Barr, cytomegalovirus,
  - infectious mononucleosis (glandular fever),
  - parasitic;
- vascular:
  - ischaemia,
  - atherosclerotic emboli,
  - lupus;
- other:
  - ectopic pregnancy,
  - ovarian cyst,

- ○ parenteral nutrition,
- ○ hypothermia,
- ○ pregnancy,
- ○ scorpion venom.
  (Sources: Hale et al., 2000; Cole, 2002; Swaroop, et al., 2004)

## Pathogenesis

Pancreatitis without parenchymal necrosis is termed interstitial or oedematous pancreatitis and is self-limiting (Cole, 2002). The most severe type – necrotising or hamorrhagic – often leads to complications and can be fatal. Whatever the cause of pancreatitis active pancreatic enzymes – trypsin, phospholipase A and elastase – are released into pancreatic tissue and cause cellular damage, cellular death, oedema and haemorrhage. If the condition remains untreated enzymes continue to be released and tissue damage (autodigestion) continues. Platelet-activating factor is released which activates the release of kinin, fibrinolysis and the complement system. These mediators contribute to tissue injury throughout the organs, leading to impairment of function (Hale et al., 2000).

## Clinical features

Clinical features of pancreatitis are notoriously variable (Taylor, 2005) and include:

- severe right upper quadrant pain: can radiate to the back and other quadrants of the abdomen. Worsens on lying down, eating a fatty meal or drinking alcohol,
- nausea and vomiting,
- diaphoresis,
- abdominal distension and guarding,
- hypotension and tachycardia,
- low-grade pyrexia,
- decreased breath sounds on auscultation,
- fever.

## Investigations

Investigations which should be undertaken include:

- serum glucose;
- urea and electrolytes;
- serum C-reactive protein (CRP): a general marker of inflammatory or infective processes.
- liver function tests
- full blood count;
- serum amylase and/or lipase;
- arterial blood gas analysis;
- chest X-ray: left-sided pleural effusion is a frequent complication of pancreatitis;
- abdominal X-ray: to determine the presence of dilated common bile duct or gallstones and eliminate other diagnosis such as perforated bowel;
- ultrasound scan of abdomen: most useful in diagnosing oedematous pancreatitis and has the advantage of being performed at the patient's bedside;
- abdominal CT scan: to detect gallstones, pancreatic necrosis, pseudocyst, abscess or eliminate pancreatitis;

## Treatment

The initial treatment of severe acute pancreatitis is supportive. Nearly half of patients with severe acute pancreatitis will have other organ dysfunction and require management by a multidisciplinary team (Swaroop et al., 2004).

- Assess the patient following the ABCDE approach described in Chapter 1. Evaluate MEWS score, alert medics/outreach if necessary (see p. 298).
- Ensure that the patient has a clear airway: if the patient has an altered conscious level, the airway is at risk. Nurse in the lateral position and consider inserting a basic airway device, such as an oropharyngeal airway, if unconscious. Consider the need for tracheal intubation.

- Administer high-flow oxygen using a non-rebreathe mask (Figure 1.4). Establish oxygen-saturation monitoring using a pulse oximeter.
- Monitor vital signs at regular intervals, including hourly urine output, respiratory rate and Early Warning Score (if used).
- Insert a wide-bore IV cannula (e.g. 14 gauge) or preferably a CVC.
- Aggressive fluid resuscitation is needed to maintain intravascular volume: this is depleted because of third-space losses (Hughes, 2004).
- Maintain electrolyte balance with the use of supplements as required.
- Commence nutrition early: evidence suggests that the enteral route is preferable to parenteral as a reduction in the length of stay, less infectious morbidity and faster recovery times have been demonstrated (McClave et al., 2006).
- Administer regular analgesia, preferably opiates.
- Administer anti-emetics for nausea and vomiting. A nasogastric tube may be necessary to decompress the stomach and prevent vomiting (Hughes, 2004).
- Prevention of infection by administering broad-spectrum antibiotics may be beneficial (Swaroop et al., 2004).
- Selective gut decontamination and the use of octreotide to reduce pancreatic enzyme secretion remain unproven (Swaroop et al., 2004; Taylor, 2005).
- Endoscopic sphincterotomy has been shown to reduce complications and mortality in severe acute pancreatitis due to biliary obstruction (Swaroop et al., 2004).
- Consider surgical debridement for infected necrosis followed by continual abdominal lavage post-operatively (Swaroop et al., 2004).

**Complications**

Complications of severe pancreatitis include:

- pancreatic necrosis;
- pancreatic pseudocyst;

- pancreatic abscess;
- sepsis;
- renal failure: due to reduced renal perfusion or micro-emboli;
- pulmonary complications, for example atelectasis or pleural effusion: due to abdominal distension and reduced diaphragm movement;
- diabetic ketoacidosis;
- hyperglycaemia due to disruption of the negative feedback mechanism;
- hypotension due to third-space fluid losses because of increased vessel permeability can progress to shock;
- tachycardia: due to compensatory mechanisms in response to reduced cardiac output;
- coagulopathy, for example disseminated intravascular coagulation and intravascular thrombi, due to the activation of pro-thrombin and plasminogen by trypsin;
- coma.

(Sources: Cole, 2002; Swaroop et al., 2004)

## GASTROINTESTINAL HAEMORRHAGE

The incidence of acute upper gastrointestinal haemorrhage (AUGIH) in the UK is approximately one per 1000 adults/year (Rockall & Northfield, 2003) and the incidence increases with age. The management of gastrointestinal haemorrhage is multidisciplinary and successful outcomes are reliant upon effective fluid resuscitation, maintenance of adequate perfusion pressure, prompt haemostasis, close monitoring of organ function and preservation of organ function (Subramanian & McCashland, 2005). Outcomes for patients with non-variceal haemorrhage compared to variceal haemorrhage are more favourable as spontaneous cessation of bleeding occurs in 90% of cases (Subramanian & McCashland, 2005). Patients with variceal haemorrhage have existing liver disease and possible other organ dysfunction, which further increases mortality.

**Causes**

- Peptic ulcer,
- oesophageal varices: secondary to portal hypertension and liver disease,
- adenocarcinoma of the stomach,
- Mallory–Weiss tear,
- benign tumours,
- vascular lesions,
- trauma,
- haemorrhagic gastritis (Hardin-Pierce, 2006).

**Clinical features**

The presentation of AUGIH can be sudden and catastrophic or more insiduous depending upon the severity and location of the bleed.

- Haematemesis: may be frank blood or 'coffee ground' vomiting,
- meleana: black tarry offensive stool, will always follow a significant bleed (Rockall & Northfield, 2003),
- hypotension and tachycardia: may precede haematemesis,
- postural hypotension,
- vasoconstriction,
- diaphoresis,
- syncope,
- shock.

**Investigations**

- Full blood count including haematocrit: most useful after volume resuscitation. Haemoglobin may fall due to haemodilution and blood loss and the urea may rise due to increased protien load presented to the gut.
- coagulation screen: most useful if pre-existing liver disease;
- liver-function tests;
- urea and electrolytes;
- upper gastrointestinal endoscopy: both diagnostic and therapeutic.

### Diagnosis

Diagnosis is predominantly made upon clinical presentation and endoscopic evaluation.

### Treatment

Treatment is aimed at restoring haemodynamic stability and haemostasis.

- Assess the patient following the ABCDE approach described in Chapter 1. Evaluate MEWS score and alert medics/outreach if necessary (see p. 298).
- Ensure that the patient has a clear airway: if the patient has an altered conscious level, the airway is at risk. Nurse in the lateral position and insert a basic airway device, such as an oropharyngeal airway, if unconscious. Consider the need for tracheal intubation.
- Administer high-flow oxygen using a non-rebreathe mask. Establish oxygen-saturation monitoring using a pulse oximeter.
- Monitor vital signs at regular intervals, including hourly urine output.
- Insert two wide-bore IV cannulae (e.g. 14 gauge) or preferably a CVC.
- Restore intravascular volume with aggressive fluid resuscitation with crystalloids and packed red cells (Box 8.1). Aim to maintain haematocrit above 30% (Subramanian & McCashland, 2005).
- Administer vasopressors to maintain cardiac output with noradrenaline (norepinephrine) being the vasoconstrictor of choice: avoid agents that have beta-2 agonist activity as they may cause splanchnic vasodilation and worsen variceal bleeds (Subramanian & McCashland, 2005).
- Upper gastrointestinal endoscopy is needed within the first 24 h of the bleed to apply haemostatic therapy where necessary, for example adrenaline or sclerosants, laser or diathermy or if this is not possible identify the position of the lesion if surgery is necessary (Subramanian & McCashland, 2005).

---

**Box 8.1 Best-practice guidelines for transfusion of blood**

Patients must have an identification (ID) band which includes the following details: last name, first name, hospital number, date of birth and gender.

ID band must be checked at the bedside against the compatibility label on the blood pack, the prescription chart and the patient's progress notes.

Preferably get the patient to confirm all of their identification verbally.

Check compatibility of blood groups with the patient's own against the blood bag and expiry date. Do not commence transfusion if any of the details do not correlate. Only administer the blood after this bedside check is completed. Two nurses (at least one should be registered) performing these checks will reduce the risk of administration error.

Ascertain whether the patient has experienced any adverse reactions to a previous transfusion.

Observe and record patient's blood pressure, pulse, temperature prior to transfusion of each unit of blood.

Temperature and pulse should be repeated 15 min following commencement of each bag; follow local guidelines after this.

Inform the patient of possible adverse reactions to the transfusion. Reassure them that these are comparatively rare.

Closely observe the patient for adverse reactions during the transfusion.

Sources: Parris and Grant-Casey (2007) and Atterbury (2001).

---

Endoscopic ligation may be performed for oesophageal varices (Atassi, 2002).

- Replace clotting factors with fresh frozen plasma and consider recombinant Factor VII (rFVIIa; this is emerging as a procoagulant that can rapidly correct severe coagulopathy).
- Surgery will be necessary if there is exsanguination and the bleeding is not amenable to endoscopy (Rockall & Northfield, 2003). Peptic ulcer haemorrhage can be catastrophic because of the close proximity to major arteries in the stomach, for example the left gastric artery. Surgical over-sewing or resection of a bleeding peptic ulcer may be necessary.

- Surgery: transjugular intrahepatic portosystemic shunting for oesophageal varices. An artificial vascular shunt is created between the systemic and portal circulation to decompress the variceal vasculature.
- Initiate balloon tamponade (Sengstaken–Blakemore tube) for compression of oesophageal varices.
- Consider an infusion of octreotide 50 µg IV bolus followed by 50 µg/h for 5 days. Octreotide indirectly inhibits the release of vasodilator hormones, causing splanchnic vasoconstriction and reduced portal inflow (Subramanian & McCashland, 2005).
- Mallory–Weiss tear (a small laceration in the mucosa at the gastroesophageal junction usually secondary to excessive vomiting) can present as a small bleed or massive haemorrhage. Bleeding may stop spontaneously but may require upper gastrointestinal endoscopy and embolisation of the bleeding vessel (Hardin-Pierce, 2006).

**Complications of AUGIH**

Complications of AUGIH include:

- shock,
- renal failure,
- coagulopathy, for example disseminated intravascular coagulation,
- acute respiratory distress syndrome,
- exsanguination.

**ACUTE LOWER GASTROINTESTINAL (LGI) HAEMORRHAGE**

The incidence of LGI bleeds has not been defined but is common in clinical practice. Most episodes of LGI haemorrhage will stop spontaneously; however, 35% will require a blood transfusion and 5% will require urgent surgical intervention (Rockall & Northfield, 2003). LGI hemorrhage is defined as bleeding from the bowel distal to the ligament of Treitz (Rana, 2004).

**Causes**

The causes of LGI haemorrhage include:

- diverticular disease (40%),
- inflammatory bowel disease, for example, Crohn's disease, ulcerative colitis or ischaemic colitis (20%),
- neoplasms (15%),
- benign ano-rectal disease (10%),
- arteriovenous malformations (2%),
- polyps,
- Meckels diverticulum,
- varices,
- generalised mucosal bleeding in the presence of coagulopathy.

(Source: Rockall & Northfield, 2003)

## Clinical features

- Passage of bright red blood per rectum (Rana, 2004),
- hypotension and tachycardia,
- postural hypotension,
- vasoconstriction,
- diaphoresis,
- syncope,
- shock.

## Investigations: diagnostic and therapeutic

- Full blood count including haematocrit: most useful after volume resuscitation;
- coagulation screen: to ascertain presence of coagulopathy;
- liver-function tests;
- urea and electrolytes;
- examination of stool: bright red blood separate from stool suggests ano-rectal disease (Rockall & Northfield, 2003);
- colonoscopy is diagnostic and also therapeutic in LGI haemorrhage. It enables the use of thermal contact modalities or aderenaline injections in cases of diverticular and vascular ectasia. Other causes of LGI bleeding can be effectively treated during colonoscopy (Rana, 2004);

- angiographic therapy: facilitates examination of the superior mesenteric artery if this is not the source of bleeding the inferior mesenteric and celiac vessels are studied. To ascertain a diagnosis with angiography active bleeding must be taking place at the time of the examination (Subramanian & McCashland, 2005). Angiographic haemostasis can be obtained by using intra-arterial vasopressin or embolisation;
- surgery: for the exsanguinating patient who has been refractory to other interventions, surgical resection will be indicated.

**Treatment**

For massive LGI haemorrhage treatment is aimed at restoring haemodynamic stability and intravascular volume.

- Assess the patient following the ABCDE approach described in Chapter 1. Evaluate MEWS score and alert medics/outreach if necessary (see p. 298).
- Ensure that the patient has a clear airway: if the patient has an altered conscious level, the airway is at risk. Nurse in the lateral position and consider inserting a basic airway device, such as an oropharyngeal airway, if unconscious. Tracheal intubation may be required.
- Administer high-flow oxygen using a non-rebreathe mask. Establish oxygen-saturation monitoring using a pulse oximeter.
- Monitor vital signs at regular intervals, including hourly urine output.
- Insert two wide-bore IV cannulae (e.g. 14 gauge) or preferably a CVC.
- Restore intravascular volume with aggressive fluid resuscitation with crystalloids and packed red cells; aim to maintain haematocrit above 30% (Subramanian & McCashland, 2005).
- Administer vasopressors as necessary to maintain cardiac output and organ perfusion.
- Proceed to therapeutic interventions as described above.

## CONCLUSION

Gastrointestinal emergencies can be sudden and catastrophic in presentation, requiring immediate and life-saving intervention. They can also present in a more insidious manner, requiring advanced assessment and clinical skills to identify and appropriately manage them to improve outcomes.

## REFERENCES

Atassi, KA (2002) Bleeding oesophageal varices. *Nursing* **32**(4), 96

Atterbury, C (2001) Blood transfusion – 4. *Nursing Times* **97**(28), 45

Cole, L (2002) Unravelling the mystery of acute pancreatitis. *Dimensions of Critical Care Nursing* **21**(3), 86–90

Day, HL & Taylor, RM (2006) The liver – part 5: acute liver failure. *Nursing Times* **102**(2), 26–7

Hale, AS, Moseley, MJ & Warner, SC (2000) Treating pancreatitis in the acute care setting. *Dimensions of Critical Care Nursing* **19**(4), 15–21

Hardin-Pierce, M (2006) Acute gastrointestinal dysfunction. In *High Acuity Nursing*, 4th edn, pp. 694–730. Pearson Education, Upper Saddle River, NJ

Hughes, E (2004) Understanding the care of patients with acute pancreatitis. *Nursing Standard* **18**(18), 45–52

Kulkarni, S & Cronin, II, DC (2005) Fulminant hepatic failure cited. In Hall, JB, Schmidt, GA & Wood, LDH (eds), *Principles of Critical Care*, 3rd edn, pp. 1279–88. McGraw-Hill, New York

Marrero, J, Martinez, FJ & Hyzy, R (2003) Advances in critical care hepatology. *American Journal of Respiratory and Critical Care Medicine* **168**(12), 1421–6

McClave, SA, Chang, W, Dhaliwal, R, *Heyland, DK* (2006) Nutritional support in acute pancreatitis: a systematic review of the literature. *Journal of Parenteral and Enteral Nutrition* **30**(2), 143–63

McGuiness, A (2007) Role of the nurse in managing patients with hepatic cerebral oedema. *British Journal of Nursing* **16**(6), 340–3

O'Neal, H, Olds, J & Webster, N (2006) Manging patients with acute liver failure: developing a tool for practitioners. *Nursing in Critical Care* **11**(2), 63–8

Parris, E & Grant-Casey, J (2007) Promoting safer blood transfusion practice in hospital. *Nursing Standard* **21**(41), 35–8

Rana, A (2004) Lower gastrointestinal bleeding. www.emedicine.com/radio/topic301.htm (accessed 11 August 2007)

Rockall, TA & Northfield, T (2003) Gastrointestinal bleeding. In Warrell, DA, Cox, TM & Firth, JD (eds), *Oxford Textbook of Medicine*, 4th edn, pp. 511–14. Oxford University Press, Oxford

Sood, G & Jones, BA (2006) Acute liver failure. www.emedicine.com/med/topic990.htm (accessed 22 August 2007)

Stadbauer, V, Krisper, P, Aigner, R, Haditsch, B, Jung, A, Lackner, C, et al. (2006) Effect of extracorporeal liver support by MARS™ and Promethius™ on serum cytokines in acute-on-chronic liver failure. *Critical Care* **10**(6), R169–76

Starr, S & Hand, H (2002) Nursing care of chronic and acute liver failure. *Nursing Standard* **16**(40), 47–54

Subramanian, R & McCashland, T (2005) Gastrointestinal haemorrhage. In Hall, JB, Schmidt, GA & Wood, LDH (eds), *Principles of Critical Care*, pp. 1261–78. McGraw-Hill, New York

Swaroop, VS, Chari, ST & Clain, JE (2004) Severe acute pancreatitis. *Journal of the American Medical Association* **291**(23), 2865–8

Taylor, BR (2005) Acute pancreatitis in the critically ill. In Hall, JB, Schmidt, GA & Wood, LDH (eds), *Principles of Critical Care*, pp. 1299–1308. McGraw-Hill, New York

Wolf, D (2007) Hepatic encephalopathy. www.emedicine.com/med/topic3185.htm (accessed 15 August 2007)

# Endocrine Emergencies

9

## Philip Jevon

### INTRODUCTION

Endocrine emergencies account for approximately 1.5% of all hospital emergency admissions in England; the majority are related to diabetes (Kearney & Dang, 2007). The other endocrine emergencies, although less common, are in some ways more important simply because of their rarity (Savage et al., 2004).

The aim of this chapter is to allow the reader to understand the treatment of endocrine emergencies.

### LEARNING OUTCOMES

At the end of this chapter the reader will be able to discuss the treatment for:

❏ diabetic ketoacidosis (DKA),
❏ hyperosmolar non-ketotic coma (HONC),
❏ hypoglycaemia,
❏ acute adrenal insufficiency,
❏ phaecromocytoma or catacholamine crisis.

### DIABETIC KETOACIDOSIS (DKA)

DKA is an acute complication of diabetes typically characterised by hyperglycaemia, ketone body formation and metabolic acidosis (Wallace & Matthews, 2004). DKA can be life-threatening; if untreated coma and death will occur (Marcovitch, 2005).

DKA remains a major contributor to morbidity and mortality in diabetes (Wallace & Matthews, 2004). Mortality rates are between 5 and 10%, and are even as high as 20% in the elderly (Boon et al., 2007; McPhee et al., 2007). Although mortality is usually due to an underlying morbidity, such as sepsis or acute coronary syndrome (Wallace & Matthews, 2004), sometimes it is due to delays in diagnosis and errors in management (Boon et al., 2007). DKA is the commonest cause of death in young persons with diabetes (National Centre for Health Statistics, 1997).

### Incidence

DKA accounted for nearly 8400 hospital admissions in England in 2004/2005 (NHS Health and Social Care Information Centre, 2007). Although it is usually associated with new cases of type 1 diabetes (Boon et al., 2007; Steinmann, 2007), it can also occur in type 2 diabetes, particularly in African-Americans and ethnic minorities (Umpierrez et al., 1999), particularly when severe stress, for example sepsis or trauma, is present (McPhee et al., 2007). Some studies suggest that up to 40% of DKA admissions are due to deliberate insulin self-manipulation.

### Pathogenesis

Severe insulin deficiency (partial or complete), together with elevated levels of circulating catecholamines and other stress hormones, lead to increased glucose production in the liver and impaired glucose uptake in the tissues (Kearney & Dang, 2007). There is increased lipolysis (fat breakdown) and ketone bodies are produced, leading to metabolic acidosis (Savage et al., 2004).

Hyperglycaemia causes a profound osmotic diuresis which leads to dehydration and loss of electrolytes, particularly sodium and potassium (Boon et al., 2007). The loss of potassium is further exacerbated by metabolic acidosis and vomiting (Boon et al., 2007).

### Causes

Causes of DKA include:

- infection: usually urinary-tract infection or pneumonia;
- newly presenting type 1 diabetes (10–20%);
- errors with insulin administration (15–30%): for example, giving the wrong dose of insulin, omitting dose(s) or failing to increase the dose during episodes of illness;
- intercurrent illnesses: for example, surgery, trauma, myocardial ischaemia or pancreatitis;

- miscellaneous (5%): for example, drugs or alcohol misuse;
- unknown (40%).

(Umpierrez & Kitabchi, 2003; Williams and Pickup, 2004):

## Clinical features

The presentation of DKA is usually within 24 h, although symptoms may be present for several days before ketoacidosis develops (Kearney & Dang, 2007). Clinical features of DKA include:

- polyuria: due to osmotic diuresis;
- polydipsia: due to osmotic diuresis;
- weight loss: due to catabolism and dehydration;
- generalised weakness;
- fruity odour on the breath: sometimes described as a pear-drop- or a nail-varnish-type of smell; this is due to ketones being excreted via the lungs (Lewis, 2000);
- Kussmaul's respirations: rapid deep breathing due to metabolic acidosis;
- nausea and vomiting (present in 50–80% of patients);
- abdominal pain (present in about 30% of cases);
- coma (present in 10% of cases).

(Palmer, 2004; Trachtenbarg, 2005;
see also Diabetes UK website, www.diabetes.org.uk)

## Investigations

Investigations that should be undertaken include:

- bedside assessment of blood glucose and blood ketones;
- routine bloods: urea and electrolytes, full blood count, glucose and bicarbonate;
- arterial blood gas analysis;
- urinalysis to detect ketonuria;
- infection screen: blood and urine cultures, C-reactive protein (CRP) and chest X-ray;
- ECG.

(Boon et al., 2007; Wyatt et al., 2006; Kearney & Dang, 2007)

**Diagnosis**

Diagnostic criteria for DKA as defined by the American Diabetes Association are (Kitabchi et al., 2004):

- blood glucose >13.8 mmol/l,
- pH <7.30,
- serum bicarbonate <18 mmol/l,
- anion gap >10,
- ketonaemia.

Hyperglycaemia, ketosis and acidosis can be diagnosed within a few minutes of the patient presenting, by measuring blood glucose and blood ketones at the bedside using a meter, and venous blood pH on a blood gas analyser (Wallace & Matthews, 2004).

Blood ketones can now be measured at the bedside, using blood from a fingerprick test and a hand-held meter device (Figure 9.1). The meter is reliable and accurate (Byrne et al., 2000). The use of blood ketone tests, rather than urine ketone tests, for diagnosis and monitoring of DKA, is now recommended by the American Diabetes Association (2004). Sometimes bedside urinalysis using a urine dipstick test can give the misleading impression that ketosis is not improving, and from a practical point of view there can be a problem obtaining urine samples from

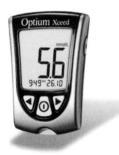

**Figure 9.1** The Optium Xceed Meter
Produced with kind permission from Abbott Diabetes Care, UK.

severely dehydrated patients at the time of presentation (Wallace & Matthews, 2004).

**Treatment**

Agreed protocols for the rapid and effective treatment of DKA by appropriately trained healthcare professionals should be agreed and available locally; these protocols should include the management of acute complications and procedures to minimise the risk of recurrence (Department of Health, 2003). It is important to follow these locally agreed policies. The key principles of the treatment of DKA will now be described.

The treatment of DKA involves careful clinical evaluation, correction of metabolic abnormalities, identification and treatment of precipitating and comorbid conditions, appropriate long-term treatment of diabetes and plans to prevent recurrence (Eledrisi et al., 2006). The priorities initially are as follows.

- Assess the patient following the ABCDE approach (Chapter 1). Evaluate MEWS score, alert medics/outreach if necessary (see p. 298).
- Ensure that the patient has a clear airway: if the patient has altered conscious level then their airway is at risk. Nurse in the lateral position and consider inserting a basic airway device, for example an oropharyngeal airway, if the patient is unconscious. Consider the need for tracheal intubation.
- Administer high-flow oxygen using a non-rebreathe mask (Figure 1.4). Establish monitoring of oxygen saturation using a pulse oximeter.
- Insert a wide-bore intravenous (IV) cannula (e.g. 14 gauge).
- Commence IV fluids: The actual rate of fluid administration will depend on the patient's clinical status; for example, in shock, the infusion rate will need to be increased. Subsequent fluid replacement would include 1000 ml of 0.9% normal saline in the first hour, followed by 500 ml/h in the next 2–3 h (Wyatt et al., 2006). It is usual to replace the fluid deficit (5–8 litres in

DKA) over a period of 24 h (Kearney & Dang, 2007). It is important to avoid rapid IV infusion in patients with cardiovascular compromise and in young patients for whom there is a risk of cerebral oedema developing (Kearney & Dang, 2007). Change to 0.45% normal saline if the plasma sodium is >150 mmol/l (Wyatt et al., 2006). The intracellular water deficit needs to be redressed using a dextrose (10%) and not a saline solution: this is done once the blood glucose levels are <15 mmol (see below) (Boon et al., 2007; Wyatt et al., 2006). The plasma glucose levels should be monitored regularly, initially at least hourly.

- Establish continuous ECG monitoring: electrolyte abnormalities, particularly hypokalaemia, can cause life-threatening cardiac arrhythmias (Resuscitation Council UK, 2006).
- Commence low-dose insulin via IV infusion (6 units/h) (other routes are possible for insulin administration, e.g. subcutaneously); once the blood sugar is <15 mmol/l, reduce the insulin infusion to 4 units/h and replace the saline infusion with 10% dextrose (Wyatt et al., 2006).
- Administer potassium 20 mmol/h via a potassium chloride solution unless the plasma potassium is >5.5 mmol; note, although total body potassium is low, plasma potassium levels may be normal, low or high (Wyatt et al., 2006). The plasma potassium levels should be monitored closely and the optimal range is 4–5 mmol/l (Kearney & Dang, 2007).
- If plasma pH <7, administer sodium bicarbonate 1.4% 500 ml over 30 min (Kearney & Dang, 2007).
- Consider inserting a nasogastric tube if the patient has an impaired level of consciousness, because of the risk of gastroparesis, vomiting/regurgitation of gastric contents and aspiration.
- Insert a urinary catheter and monitor urine output closely.
- Consider broad-spectrum antibiotics if an infection is suspected; pyrexia is rarely present and an increase in white cell count could just be due to ketonaemia (Wyatt et al., 2006).

- Consider inserting a central venous catheter to monitor central venous pressure (e.g. in critical illness).
- Monitor the patient's vital signs closely: fluid balance, blood glucose, blood ketones, arterial blood gases, and urea and electrolytes. The American Diabetes Association recommends the following criteria for the resolution of DKA: blood glucose <11 mmol/l, venous bicarbonate >18 mmol/l and venous pH >7.30 (Kearney & Dang, 2007).
- Involve the diabetes team at the earliest opportunity; for example, making the decision to stop continuous IV infusion of insulin in favour of subcutaneous injections of insulin is best made by senior experienced medical staff (Kearney & Dang, 2007). Appropriate on-going care is essential.
- Arrange for appropriate referral to the diabetes nurse specialist (Department of Health, 2003); patient education is important as 50% of DKA admissions are preventable (Kearney & Dang, 2007).

### Complications of DKA

Complications of DKA include:

- cerebral oedema: causes include rapid reduction of blood glucose and use of hypotonic fluids and/or bicarbonate;
- acute respiratory distress syndrome;
- deep-vein thrombosis and pulmonary embolism (hyperglycaemia causes a hypercoagulable state);
- acute left ventricular failure: due to rapid IV infusion of fluids.
                    (Boon et al., 2007; Wyatt et al., 2006)

## HYPEROSMOLAR NON-KETOTIC COMA (HONC)

HONC develops over days or weeks and is caused by inadequacy of insulin resulting in severe hyperglycaemia (>33.3 mmol/l) (Kearney & Dang, 2007). In 2004–2005 HONC accounted for approximately 2000 hospital admissions (NHS Health and Social Care Information Centre, 2007). Mortality is high (15%), particularly in the elderly.

### Causes

Infection is the most common cause of HONC; other causes include stressful events such as stroke, myocardial infarction and surgery (Kearney & Dang, 2007).

### Pathogenesis

The pathogenesis of HONC is similar to that of DKA (see above), except that the patient does not develop ketoacidosis (Kearney & Dang, 2007).

### Investigations

As for DKA: see above.

### Diagnosis

Diagnostic criteria for HONC as defined by the American Diabetes Association are (Kitabchi et al., 2004):

- blood glucose >33.3 mmol/l,
- pH >7.30,
- serum bicarbonate >15 mmol/l,
- serum osmolality >320,
- trace of ketones in the urine.

### Treatment

As for DKA: see above.

### HYPOGLYCAEMIA

Hypoglycaemia is defined as a blood glucose level <4 mmol/l (www.diabetes.org.uk). It can mimic any neurological presentation including alert conscious level, seizures, acute confusion or isolated hemiparesis. Therefore it is important to always exclude hypoglycaemia in any patient with the above.

The risks of hazard from hypoglycaemia are small (Watkins, 2003), although altered consciousness can lead to airway compromise. A prolonged severe hypoglycaemic episode can cause moderate to severe neuropsychological impairments (Kubiak et al.,

2004). Hypoglycaemia can cause an acute cerebral injury, causing hemiplegia (Shirayama et al., 2004).

### Incidence

The exact incidence of hypoglycaemic episodes is unknown, as most are treated successfully at home and some, particularly those occurring at night, may not be recognised (Appleton & Jerreat, 1995). On average there are over 90,000 calls to the emergency services each year for hypoglycaemia (Sampson et al., 2006). In 2004/2005 there were 8000 admissions to hospital in England due to hypoglycaemia (Kearney & Dang, 2007).

### Causes

Common causes of hypoglycaemia include:

- too much insulin,
- delayed or missed meal or snack,
- not enough food, especially carbohydrate,
- unplanned or strenuous exercise,
- alcohol consumption without food,
- idiopathy.

(www.diabetes.org.uk)

Although most hypoglycaemic episodes occur in patients on insulin treatment, some occur in those on sulphonylurea drugs (Shorr et al., 1997). Alcohol intake can cause hypoglycaemia several hours later; the effects of alcohol may also mask hypoglycaemic symptoms (Appleton & Jerreat, 1995).

Medical causes of hypoglycaemia include:

- liver failure,
- Addison's disease,
- pituitary insufficiency.

(Wyatt et al., 2006).

### Clinical features

The clinical features of hypoglycaemia vary from person to person, although they are often constant for an individual (www.

diabetes.org.uk). Individuals may recognise different symptoms and these may change as the duration of diabetes increases (McLaren & Somerville, 1988).

Clinical features of hypoglycaemia can be classified as either autonomic (usually present first when the blood glucose is 3.3–3.6 mmol/l) or related to neuroglycopenia (usually present when the blood glucose is <2.6 mmol/l):

- autonomic: sweating, hunger, hot sensation, anxiety, nausea and vomiting;
- neuroglycopenia: fatigue, visual disturbance, unco-ordinated and altered behaviour, drowsiness, confusion and, if untreated, convulsions and coma.

(Kearney & Dang, 2007; www.diabetes.org.uk)

Note that in patients with chronic hyperglycaemia, the autonomic clinical features may be triggered at higher blood glucose levels (Boyle et al., 1988).

The patient is usually aware that hypoglycaemia is developing (www.diabetes.org.uk), although this may not always be the case. In addition, recurrent hypoglycaemic episodes can lead to diminished patient awareness of impending hypoglycaemia (Watkins, 2003; Kearney and Dang, 2007). The nurse should therefore be alert to the clinical features of hypoglycaemia.

### Investigations

Bedside blood glucose measurement should be undertaken, and a blood sample should be sent to the laboratory.

### Diagnosis

The biomedical diagnosis of hypoglycaemia is a blood sugar <2.5 mmol/l (Kearney & Dang, 2007).

### Treatment

- Assess the patient following the ABCDE approach described in Chapter 1. Evaluate MEWS score, alert medics/outreach if necessary (see p. 298). Treatment will depend on the patient's conscious level and degree of co-operation (Wyatt et al., 2006).

- If the patient's conscious levels allows safe eating and drinking, offer the simplest available carbohydrate-containing food that can be absorbed quickly, for example sugary foods, a glass of lucozade or cola (not diet drinks), a glass of fruit juice, or three or more glucose tablets (www.diabetes.org.uk). This can then be followed by long-acting carbohydrates, for example digestive biscuits (Kearney & Dang, 2007).

- In some clinical settings, GlucoGel® (formally known as Hypo-stop; a dextrose gel, rapidly absorbed via the buccal mucosa) may be administered (BMA & Royal Pharmaceutical Society of GB, 2007; Kearney & Dang, 2007).

- If the patient's conscious level has deteriorated, ensure the airway is clear and maintained; place the patient in the lateral position. If they are unconscious consider inserting a basic airway device; for example, an oropharyngeal airway.

- Administer high-flow oxygen using a non-rebreathe mask (Figure 1.4). Establish monitoring of oxygen saturation using a pulse oximeter.

- Insert a wide-bore IV cannula (e.g. 14 gauge).

- Administer 25–50 ml of 50% dextrose followed by a 0.9% normal saline flush (50% glucose solution is hypertonic and causes thrombophlebitis) (Wyatt et al., 2006). The solution is very viscous, making it difficult to draw up (use a quill) and to administer. Glucose solutions of 10 and 20% can also be used, but larger volumes will be required (BMA & Royal Pharmaceutical Society of GB, 2007).

- If there is difficulty securing IV access (Wyatt et al., 2006), administer glucagon 1 mg intramuscularly. Glucagon, the hormone produced by the A cells of the islets in the pancreas, increases the blood glucose level by mobilising glycogen stores in the liver (Watkins, 2003). The majority of people with type 1 diabetes lose their glucagon response to hypoglycaemia within 5 years of diagnosis (Bolli et al., 1983). The recommended dose for glucagon is 1 mg subcutaneously, intramuscularly or intravenously (BMA & Royal Pharmaceutical Society of GB, 2007).

- Monitor the patient's response and conscious level. Ninety per cent of patients will recover fully in 20 min (Wyatt et al., 2006).
- Try to establish the possible cause of the hypoglycaemia. To prevent a repeat hypoglycaemic episode, offer the patient food that contains starchy carbohydrates (absorbed more slowly); for example, a sandwich, fruit, a bowl of cereal or biscuits and milk (www.diabetes.org.uk).
- Educate the patient. Education is the key to preventing recurrent or severe hypoglycaemia (Chelliah & Burge, 2004). It may be necessary to involve the diabetes team.
- Reassure the patient. Repeated episodes of hypoglycaemia may cause extreme emotional distress, even when the episodes are relatively mild (Chelliah & Burge, 2004).

## ACUTE ADRENAL INSUFFICIENCY

Acute adrenal insufficiency is a potentially fatal condition resulting from inadequate secretion of cortisol and/or aldosterone (Boon et al., 2007).

It should be suspected in patients who present with unexplained fatigue, hyponatraemia or hypotension (Boon et al., 2007).

### Causes

Adrenal insufficiency can result from a primary or secondary cause:

- primary adrenal insufficiency results from adrenal damage, for example Addison's disease;
- secondary adrenal insufficiency results from adrenocorticotrophic hormone (ACTH) deficiency due to pituitary or hypothalamic damage;
- abrupt withdrawal of therapeutic steroid therapy can also cause ACTH deficiency.

(Leach, 2004)

Acute adrenal insufficiency can be precipitated by stress – for example from trauma or surgery – or may be seen in patients with undiagnosed chronic adrenal insufficiency or following stress in sepsis or adrenal haemorrhage during critical illness (Leach, 2004).

## Clinical features

Clinical features include:

- shock, for example hypotension, tachycardia and pallor,
- anorexia,
- nausea and vomiting,
- abdominal pain,
- pyrexia,
- fatigue and lethargy.

(Kearney & Dang, 2007)

## Treatment

- Assess the patient following the ABCDE approach described in Chapter 1. Evaluate MEWS score, alert medics/outreach if necessary (see p. 298).
- Administer high-flow oxygen using a non-rebreathe mask (Figure 1.4). Establish monitoring of oxygen saturation using a pulse oximeter.
- Insert a wide-bore IV cannula (e.g. 14 gauge).
- Administer 2–3 litres 0.9% normal saline IV. Sometimes aggressive fluid therapy (e.g. 6 litres over 24 h) and inotropic support are required (Leach, 2004).
- Administer hydrocortisone 100 mg IV every 6 h for 24 h, followed by 100 mg IV every 8 h for the next 24 h; the dose can then be adjusted according to the clinical picture (McPhee et al., 2007).
- Administer fludrocortisone 30–300 µg orally per day (BMA & Royal Pharmaceutical Society of GB, 2007), titrating the dose according to the patient's symptoms and postural blood pressure (Kearney & Dang, 2007).
- Obtain sputum and urine specimens for culture. Commence appropriate antibiotics if necessary.
- Identify and treat the precipitating cause of the adrenal insufficiency.

## PHAEOCHROMOCYTOMA OR CATECHOLAMINE CRISIS

Phaeochromocytoma or catecholamine crisis is a small catechol-amine-producing tumour, usually involving one or more of the adrenal glands, which can lead to uncontrolled and irregular secretion of the hormones adrenaline or noradrenaline (McFerran & Martin, 2003; Ramrakha & Moore, 2004). It can lead to extreme hypertension; a systolic blood pressure of >220 mmHg and a diastolic blood pressure of >120 mmHg require emergency treatment (Kearney & Dang, 2007).

### Causes

Hypertensive or catecholamine crisis can be triggered by straining, exercise, surgery, pressure on the abdomen and drugs, for example opiates and anaesthesics (Ramrakha & Moore, 2004; Kearney & Dang, 2007).

### Pathogenesis

A small catecholamine-producing tumour of either one or both adrenal glands leads to uncontrolled and irregular secretion of the hormones adrenaline or noradrenaline, which can cause extreme hypertension.

### Clinical features

Clinical features can include:

- hypertension,
- headache,
- profound sweating,
- pallor,
- significant tachycardia,
- palpitations,
- numbness, tingling and coolness at the peripheries.
  (Ram, 1988; Ramrakha & Moore, 2004; Kearney & Dang, 2007)

### Investigations

There are no specific investigations to diagnose phaeochromocytoma acutely (Ramrakha & Moore, 2004), 24 hour catecholamine collection could be considered.

**Diagnosis**

It is difficult to diagnose phaecochromocytoma as the cause of hypertension (Cryer, 2001). However, the classic triad of headache, palpitations and sweating in the presence of hypertension almost confirms the diagnosis (Kearney & Dang, 2007). 24 hour urine collection may be helpful.

**Treatment**

- Assess the patient following the ABCDE approach described in Chapter 1. Evaluate MEWS score, alert medics/outreach if necessary (see p. 298).
- Administer high-flow oxygen using a non-rebreamast. Establish monitoring of oxygen saturation using a pulse oximeter.
- Commence ECG monitoring and report any cardiac arrhythmias.
- Establish IV access.
- To treat hypertensive episodes, commence an IV alpha-blocker, for example phentolamine 1–5 mg every 15 min as required or phenoxybenzamine 1 mg/kg infused over a minimum of 2 h (Kearney & Dang, 2007). Although a beta-blocker may also be prescribed, it can lead to increased alpha-receptor-mediated vasoconstriction, resulting in the worsening of existing hypertension; a beta-blocker should therefore only be administered following an alpha-blocker (Kearney & Dang, 2007).
- Monitor the patient's vital signs closely, particularly blood pressure.
- Ask the patient to rest. Sometimes bed rest is indicated.
- Once blood pressure has been controlled, the definitive treatment is surgery, which is successful at controlling the blood pressure in 75% of cases (Kearney & Dang, 2007).

**Complications**

Complications of severe hypertension include vascular injuries of the brain, kidneys and eyes.

CONCLUSION

Endocrine emergencies are rare and can be life-threatening. It is important to understand the treatment of endocrine emergencies, which should not be delayed while awaiting results from investigations (Kearney & Dang, 2007). In this chapter the treatment of endocrine emergencies has been discussed.

## REFERENCES

American Diabetes Association (2004) Clinical practice recommendations 2004. *Diabetes Care* **27** (suppl 1), S94–102.

Appleton, M & Jerreat, L (1995) Hypoglycaemia. *Nursing Standard* **10**(5), 36–42

BMA & Royal Pharmaceutical Society of GB (2007) *British National Formulary 53*. BMJ Publishing, London

Bolli, G, de Feo, P, Compagnucci, P, Cartechini, MG, Angeletti, G, Santeusanio, F, Brunetti, P & Gerich, JE (1983) Abnormal glucose counterregulation in insulin-dependent diabetes mellitus. Interaction of anti-insulin antibodies and impaired glucagon and epinephrine secretion. *Diabetes* **32**, 134–41

Boon, N, Colledge, N, Walker, B & Hunter, J (2007) *Davidson's Principles & Practice of Medicine*, 20th edn. Churchill Livingstone, Edinburgh

Boyle, P, Schwartz, N, Shah, S, et al. (1988) Plasma glucose concentrations at the onset of hypoglycaemic symptoms in patients with poorly controlled diabetes and in non-diabetics. *New England Journal of Medicine* **318**, 1487–92

Byrne, H, Tieszen, K, Hollis, S, et al. (2000) Evaluation of an electrochemical sensor for measuring blood ketones. *Diabetes Care* **23**, 500–3

Chelliah, A & Burge, MR (2004) Hypoglycaemia in elderly patients with diabetes mellitus: causes and strategies for prevention. *Drugs & Aging* **21**(8), 511–30

Cryer, P (2001) Diseases of the sympathochromaffin system. In Felig P, Frohman L (eds), *Endocrinology and Metabolism*, pp. 525–51. McGraw-Hill, New York

Department of Health (2003) *National Service Framework for Diabetes*. Department of Health, London

Eledrisi, M, Alshanti, M, Shah, M, et al. (2006) Overview of the diagnosis and management of diabetic ketoacidosis. *American Journal of the Medical Sciences* **331**(5), 243–51

Kearney, T & Dang, C (2007) Diabetic and endocrine emergencies. *Postgraduate Medical Journal* **83**(976), 79–86

Kitabchi, A, Umpierrez, G, Murphy, M, et al. (2004) Hyperglycemic crisis in diabetes. *Diabetes Care* **27** (suppl 1): S94–102

Kubiak, T, Hermanns, N, Schreckling, H, Kulzer, B & Haak, T (2004) Assessment of hypoglycaemia awareness using continuous glucose monitoring. *Diabetic Medicine* **21**, 487–90

Leach, R (2004) *Critical Care Medicine at a Glance*. Blackwell Publishing, Oxford

Lewis, R (2000) Diabetic emergencies: Part 2. Hyperglycaemia. *Accident and Emergency Nursing* **8**(1), 24–30

Marcovitch, H (2005) *Black's Medical Dictionary*, 41st edn. A & C Black, London

McFerran, T & Martin, E (2003) *Minidictionary for Nurses*, 5th edn. Oxford University Press, Oxford

McLaren, E & Somerville, J (1988) Early warning signs of hypoglycaemia in ambulant diabetics. *Practical Diabetes* **5**(5), 207–8

McPhee, S, Papadakis, M & Tierney, L (2007) *Current Medical Diagnosis and Treatment*, 46th edn. McGraw Hill, London

National Centre for Health Statistics (1997) Detailed diagnosis and procedures: national discharge summary. *Vital Health Statistics* **13**, 130

NHS Health and Social Care Information Centre (2007) www.hesonline.nhs.uk (accessed 15 March 2007)

Palmer, R (2004) An overview of diabetic ketoacidosis. *Nursing Standard* **19**(10), 42–5

Ram, C (1988) Pheochromocytoma. *Cardiology Clinics* **6**, 517–35

Ramrakha, P & Moore, K (2004) *Oxford Handbook of Acute Medicine*, 2nd edn. Oxford University Press, Oxford

Resuscitation Council UK (2006) *Advanced Life Support*, 5th edn. Resuscitation Council UK, London

Sampson, M, Mortley, S & Aldridge, V (2006) The East Anglian Ambulance Trust diabetes emergencies audit-numbers and demographics. *Diabetes Medicine* **23**, 101

Savage, M, Mah, P, Weetman, A & Newell-Price, J (2004) Endocrine emergencies. *Postgraduate Medical Journal* **80**, 506–15

Shirayama, H, Ohshiro, Y, Kinjo, Y, Taira, S, Teruya, I, Nakachi, K, et al. (2004) Acute brain injury in hypoglycaemia-induced hemiplegia. *Diabetic Medicine* **21**(6), 623–4

Shorr, R, Ray, W, Daugherty, J, et al. (1997) Incidence and risk factors for serious hypoglycaemia in older persons using insulin or sulfonylureas. *Archives of Internal Medicine* **157**, 1681–6

Steinmann, R (2007) Pediatric diabetic ketoacidosis. *American Journal of Nursing* **107**(3), 72CC–72KK

Trachtenbarg, D (2005) Diabetic ketoacidosis. *American Family Physician* **71**(9), 1705–15

Umpierrez, G & Kitabchi, A (2003) Diabetic ketoacidosis: risk factors and management strategies. *Treatments in Endocrinology* **2**(2), 95–108

Umpierrez, G, Woo, W, Hagopian, W, et al. (1999) Immunogenetic analysis suggests different pathogenesis for obese and lean African-Americans with diabetic ketoacidosis. *Diabetes Care* **22**, 1517–23

Wallace, T & Matthews, D (2004) Recent advances in the monitoring and management of diabetic ketoacidosis *Quarterly Journal of Medicine* **97**, 773–80

Watkins, P (2003) *ABC of Diabetes*, 5th edn. BMJ Books, London

Williams, G & Pickup, J (2004) *Handbook of Diabetes*, 3rd edn. Blackwell Science, Oxford

Wyatt, J, Illingworth, R, Graham, C, Clancy, M & Robertson, C (2006) *Oxford Handbook of Emergency Medicine*, 3rd edn. Oxford University Press, Oxford

# Poisoning

# 10

## James Bethel

## INTRODUCTION

Poisoning can be deliberate (self-harm), accidental (unintentional) or associated with substance abuse. In the UK, paracetamol is the commonest cause of poisoning and is associated with relatively high mortality rates (Kapur et al., 2002; Schmidt & Dalhoff, 2002; Gunnell et al., 2004). Patients who take a cocktail of different drugs, and/or who take them with alcohol, are at greater risk of death than those who take a single drug (Preti et al., 2002; Schmidt & Dalhoff, 2002).

Regardless of the cause of poisoning, the priorities of treatment initially are supportive, following the ABCDE assessment outlined in Chapter 1; it is essential that the patient has a clear airway, adequate breathing and adequate circulation. The vital signs must be closely monitored, with specific attention to the drug(s) or substance(s) involved and the associated adverse side effects. Respiratory depression and cardiovascular instability are common findings associated with poisoning.

The aim of this chapter is to allow the reader to understand the medical treatment of poisoning.

## LEARNING OUTCOMES

At the end of this chapter the reader will be able to:

❏ outline the incidence and demographic pattern of poisoning,
❏ state the general treatment of poisoning,
❏ discuss psychological assessment and care,
❏ discuss the treatment of specific drugs commonly associated with poisoning.

## INCIDENCE AND DEMOGRAPHIC PATTERN OF POISONING

The UK has one of the highest rates of self-harm in Europe at 400 patients per 100,000 of the population (Horrocks, 2002); 170,000 people per annum attend for care related to self-harm (Kapur et al., 1998), mainly due to drug poisoning (overdose). Some 1176 people died of drug poisoning in the UK between 1997 and 1999 (Gunnell et al., 2004).

Demographically, the highest incidence of overdose in the UK is among young females aged 15–19 years (Samaritans, 2005), although rates of suicide are highest amongst males (Office for National Statistics, 2007). In the UK in 2005:

- 17.5 per 100,000 men committed suicide (this figure is decreasing),
- 5.8 per 100,000 women committed suicide (static),
- there were 5671 suicides among adults.

(Office for National Statistics, 2007)

In 2000 the international suicide rate was highest in Belarus (73.1 per 100,000 adults) and Lithuania (91.7 per 100,000 adults) and lowest in the Caribbean, South America and the Middle East; in Kuwait the rate was only 3.2 per 100,000 adults (World Health Organization, 2003).

Monday has the highest incidence of suicide (Office for National Statistics, 2005); deliberate self-harm by overdose is more prevalent among those who have recently been released from prison (Singleton et al., 2003) and (whether deliberate or accidental in nature) among socio-economically disadvantaged communities (Galea et al., 2003).

## GENERAL TREATMENT OF POISONING

Patients who take an overdose may present to the emergency department in a number of ways. Some will seek help immediately and may arrive either in an ambulance, with the help of their family or carers, or on their own; others may not seek help for hours or even days. Even though patients may have referred themselves for care, they may be unco-operative and unwilling to comply with assessment and treatment regimes. This could be due to guilt and shame, which has been found to be prevalent among these patients (Mayo Foundation for Medical Health and Research, 2006), or the low self-esteem that often precipitates self-injurious behaviour (Laye-Gindhu & Schonert-Reichl, 2005; Hume & Platt, 2007).

The general treatment of patients with poisoning will now be described. For details concerning the treatment of specific poisoning, see below.

- Ensure that it is safe to approach and treat the patient. With some poisons it will be necessary to take precautions to prevent self-poisoning, e.g. paraquat poisoning.
- Assess the patient following the ABCDE approach described in Chapter 1. Evaluate MEWS score, alert medics/outreach if necessary (see p. 298).
- Ensure that the patient has a clear airway. Altered consciousness, a common complication of poisoning, can lead to airway compromise. Nurse in the lateral position to minimise the risk of aspiration should vomiting or regurgitation of gastric contents occur (Wyatt et al., 2006); if the patient is unconscious, insert a basic airway device such as an oropharyngeal airway; a cuffed tracheal tube may need to be inserted to protect the airway.
- Administer high-flow oxygen using a non-rebreathe mask (Figure 1.4). Establish oxygen-saturation monitoring using a pulse oximeter. Respiratory depression is a common complication of poisoning; regular arterial blood gas analysis may be required. Where respiratory status is compromised, evidenced by apnoea, bradypnoea, low oximetry values and altered level of consciousness, then provide respiratory support; positive-pressure ventilation may be required.
- Insert a wide-bore intravenous (IV) cannula (e.g. 14 gauge). Obtain blood sample for relevant investigations including full blood count, urea and electrolytes, liver-function tests, glucose and toxic screen. Normal values of key blood tests are detailed in Box 10.1.

**Box 10.1 Normal blood values**

**Urea and electrolytes**

| | |
|---|---|
| Sodium | 132–142 mmol/l |
| Potassium | 3.4–5 mmol/l |
| Bicarbonate | 22–30 mmol/l |
| Glucose | 3.5–7 mmol/l |
| Urea | <7.5 mmol/l |

**Liver-function tests**

| | |
|---|---|
| Total protein | 63–83 g/l |
| Albumin | 30–44 g/l |
| Bilirubin | 2–17 μmol/l |
| Alkaline phosphatase | 30–135 units/l |
| Alanine aminotranferase | 7–40 units/l |
| Total calcium | 2.2–2.6 mmol/l |
| Ionised calcium | 1.18–1.30 mmol/l |
| Phosphate | 0.8–1.4 mmol/l |
| Zinc | 12–23 μmol/l |
| Magnesium | 0.7–1.0 mmol/l |

**Normal arterial blood gas values**

| | |
|---|---|
| Hydrogen ion | 36–45 mmol/l |
| pH | 7.36–7.44 |
| $pCO_2$ | 4.7–6 kPa |
| $pO_2$ | 9.3–14 kPa |
| Base excess | ±2.5 mmol/l |
| Standard bicarbonate | 21–25 mmol/l |

- Hypotension can complicate poisoning: commence IV fluids.
- Establish continuous ECG monitoring: cardiac arrhythmias can complicate poisoning;
- Consider inserting a nasogastric tube if the patient has impaired conscious level. This is because of the risk of gastroparesis, vomiting/regurgitation of gastric contents and aspiration.
- Monitor the patient's level of consciousness using AVPU and the Glasgow Coma Scale (GCS; see Chapter 6); undertake regular pupillary assessment.
- Perform bedside measurement of blood glucose; correct hypoglycaemia.

- Check the patient for injuries; important injury and illness may be masked by drugs and/or alcohol.
- Try to establish the exact cause of the poisoning; some drugs, if identified, have antidote medications which will minimise toxic side effects in overdose. It may be possible to identify tablets using MIMMS Colour Index or descriptions detailed in the *British National Formulary*.
- Seek advice concerning specific treatment and management options. Antidotes are only available for a few drugs, although they are not always necessary; TOXBASE and Poisons Information Centres can provide advice (Wyatt et al., 2006).
- Try to establish when the overdose was taken; options for treatment vary according to length of time following ingestion. Methods to reduce absorption of the drug include the following.
  - Activated charcoal: may be beneficial for patients who present within 1 h of ingestion and in some patients after this time (Wyatt et al., 2006).
  - Gastric lavage (rarely used): this may be beneficial for patients who present within 1 h of ingestion and who have not taken a caustic substance (Goldsack et al., 1999; Resuscitation Council UK, 2006); complications include hypoxia, aspiration pneumonia and oesophageal perforation (Wyatt et al., 2006).
- In patients who present some time after overdose, treatment will be aimed at treating specific toxicological side effects rather than attempting to reduce the absorption of the drug.

## PSYCHOLOGICAL ASSESSMENT AND CARE

### Importance

There is a strong association between self-harm and suicide; the incidence of suicide following an episode of self-harm is between 0.5% and 2% (Owens et al., 2002). Emergency department staff do not always have sufficient skills and knowledge to make an assessment of suicidal intent (Arbuthnot & Gillespie, 2005; Farmer & Bethel, 2006).

It is recommended that all patients presenting with deliberate self-harm receive specialist assessment (Royal College of Psychiatrists, 1994; Department of Health, 1999); unfortunately fewer than half receive this assessment and psychosocial support is poor (Kapur et al., 2002; Arbuthnot & Gillespie, 2005). It is paramount to ensure appropriate and timely referral for specialist psychological assessment following local protocols.

### Information required
When assessing the suicidal intent of the patient, it is important to establish:

- the patient's perception of the lethality of the overdose (which may be different to its actual lethality);
- whether or not the patient expected to be discovered;
- how much planning had been involved in the overdose;
- the social circumstances of the patient, for example employment status, any marital problems and whether or not there has been a recent death of a loved one.
- extent of regular substance misuse.

### SAD PERSONS score
Attempts have been made to develop assessment tools for use in patients who have self-harmed in order to gauge their suicidal intent, for example the SAD PERSONS score (Hockberger & Rothstein, 1988):

**S**ex: 1 if patient is male, 0 if female,
**A**ge: 1 if patient is under 19 or over 45,
**D**epression: 1 if present
**P**revious attempt: 1 if present,
**E**thanol abuse: 1 if present,
**R**ational thinking loss: 1 if patient is psychotic for any reason (schizophrenia, affective illness, organic brain syndrome),
**S**ocial support lacking: 1 if these are lacking, especially with recent loss of a significant other,

Organized plan: 1 if plan made and method lethal,

No spouse: 1 if divorced, widowed, separated or single (for males),

Sickness: 1 especially if chronic, debilitating, severe (e.g. non-localized cancer, epilepsy, multiple sclerosis, gastrointestinal disorders).

The scoring for this is a follows:

0–2: little risk,

3–4: follow the patient closely,

5–6: strongly consider admission,

7–10: very high risk: admit, if necessary under a section of the Mental Health Act 1983.

Patients who deliberately ingest overdoses of medication in an attempt to harm themselves have complex care needs: they will require an assessment of their psychosocial needs in addition to the assessment and management of the toxicity that may be associated with the medication they have taken. This chapter will focus on the latter aspect of care.

### Negative attitudes of healthcare staff

Negative attitudes of heathcare staff towards those who deliberately self-harm can exacerbate the challenges associated with managing such situations (McAllister et al., 2002; NICE, 2004; Mackay & Barrowclough, 2005). Such attitudes manifest as judgementalism concerning the deservedness of care, the withholding of certain aspects of care (i.e. analgesia) and a compounding of the patient's guilt by the adoption of an attitude designed to make the patient feel that they are wasting the time and resources of the department.

The adoption of a negative or judgemental attitude has indeed been found by some authors to contribute to their future suicide and staff should ensure an empathetic approach to such patients.

## TREATMENT OF SPECIFIC DRUGS COMMONLY ASSOCIATED WITH POISONING

### Paracetamol poisoning

Paracetamol became available in the UK in 1956. In 1998 the pack size of paracetamol was restricted to 16 because of concerns about the incidence of overdosage. There is some evidence that this intervention has reduced the number of paracetamol overdoses (Hawton, 2001). Some authors advocate the re-classification of paracetamol to a prescription-only medicine because of similar concerns about its toxicity in overdosage (Farley et al., 2005).

In history-taking the pattern of ingestion needs to be established as this will determine treatment. A patient who has ingested paracetamol in toxic quantities and in a staggered fashion over a long period of time will present difficulties when attempting to assess plasma concentration of the drug. In such circumstances, where the total dose is thought to exceed 150 mg/kg of body weight or 12 g (whichever is the smaller), then antidotal treatment should be instituted (Hartley, 2002). A single episode of ingestion of a toxic quantity of paracetamol, where the time of ingestion can be established, makes assessment less complicated: plasma levels of paracetamol peak at 4 h after ingestion and blood should therefore be sampled at this point and treatment based on toxicology results from this.

### Side effects

Paracetamol can cause severe liver damage if 12 g (24 tablets) or 150 mg/kg are ingested (Wyatt et al., 2006). High-risk individuals, for example alcoholics and previous overdose of paracetamol, are more susceptible to hepatic toxicity and may experience toxicity at concentrations as low as 75 mg/kg (Hartley, 2002; BMJ Clinical Evidence, 2006). Other side effects are related to hepatotoxicity, for example prolonged clotting times and hypoglycaemia (Wyatt et al., 2006). Abdominal pain, nausea and vomiting are common within the first few hours, although they may not become apparent until after 24 h; after 12 h tenderness and pain over the liver may be evident (Wyatt et al., 2006); at 3–5 days jaundice, renal failure, encephalopathy and coma may develop depending upon the quantity ingested.

### Specific investigations

Investigations should include liver-function tests (which may be normal until >18 h) and a clotting screen (prothrombin time and international normalised ratio). A prolonged international normalised ratio at >24 h is the most sensitive laboratory evidence of liver damage (Wyatt et al., 2006). Blood glucose, creatinine, arterial blood gas analysis and paracetamol levels should also be tested.

### Treatment

Administration of activated charcoal to decontaminate the gut is indicated in patients who present within 1 h of ingestion. Antidotal treatment is IV acetylcysteine (Parvolex®); this is most effective in minimising hepatotoxicity when administered within 8 h of ingestion although some therapeutic benefit has been found in administration up to 24 h following ingestion (Parker, 1990). Where patients present more than 8 h after ingestion, antidotal treatment should be instituted immediately without waiting for plasma concentration to be estimated. The recommended dose of acetylcysteine in adults is:

- 150 mg/kg of body weight in 200 ml of 5% dextrose IV over 15 min, then
- 50 mg/kg IV in 500 ml of 5% dextrose over 4 h and then
- 100 mg/kg IV in 1 litre of 5% dextrose over 16 h.

(Wyatt et al., 2006)

Methionine is an alternative antidotal treatment to acetylcysteine. Rarely used, it can be considered if the patient refuses IV treatment, if acetylcysteine is not available (Wyatt et al., 2006) or if the patient is known to be hypersensitive (allergic) to acetylcysteine. As it can exacerbate hepatotoxicity, it should not be administered more than 12 h after ingestion (Hartley, 2002). The dose is 2.5 g orally every 4 h up to a total of 10 g; it may be ineffective if the patient has been treated with activated charcoal (Wyatt et al., 2006).

### Criteria for referral to a liver transplant unit

Liver transplantation may occasionally be required if the patient presented late or was treated late; suggested transplant criteria include:

- prothrombin time >100 s,
- elevated plasma creatinine,
- hypoglycaemia,
- persistent acidosis,
- hypotension.

(Sources: Hartley, 2002; Wyatt et al., 2006)

### Aspirin poisoning

Aspirin, an analgesic and anti-pyretic drug, is also used therapeutically in the prevention of cardiovascular disease because of its anti-clotting properties. In overdose it carries a high morbidity and mortality rate.

Delays in absorption and the fact that many aspirin preparations are now enteric-coated to avoid gastric irritation mean that aspirin taken in overdose may not peak, in terms of its plasma concentration, for up to 24 h. A careful history should be taken to establish when the drug was ingested and the amount taken. Poisoning is associated with plasma concentrations of >350 mg/l and death is more common in concentrations of 700 mg/l or more (Medicines and Healthcare Products Regulatory Agency, 2005). Following the initial metabolism of aspirin, salicylic acid is produced, and it is this substance that is measured in the plasma concentration.

### Specific investigations

Investigations should include arterial blood gas analysis, glucose, urea and electrolytes, creatinine (renal function) and urinalysis. Due to the potential delay in peak plasma concentrations of salicylate being evident serial estimates of salicylate levels should be undertaken at 2- or 3-hourly intervals to ensure that plasma concentrations are falling rather than rising.

### Side effects
Common side effects include vomiting, tinnitus, vertigo, sweating, warm extremities and hyperventilation; patients may therefore present with a respiratory alkalosis compensated for by a metabolic acidosis with arterial pH being normal or slightly elevated (Kamanyire, 2002). Less common features associated with severe poisoning and/or delayed presentation include confusion, coma, hypokalaemia, pyrexia and convulsions.

### Treatment
Activated charcoal may be useful in decontaminating the gut and reducing absorption; serial doses may be administered as delays in absorption are sometimes associated with enteric-coated preparations of aspirin. Sodium bicarbonate 500 ml 1.26% IV is administered hourly for 3 h to alkalinise the urine (more effective than a massive diuresis to eliminate salicylate); urine pH should be >7.5, ideally 8.0–8.5 (Wyatt et al., 2006). In the presence of hypokalaemia, urinary alkalinity is compromised (Kamanyire, 2002; Medical and Healthcare Products Regulatory Agency, 2005); administer potassium supplements as required.

In severe poisoning (central nervous system (CNS) features, acidosis or salicylate >700 mg/l), which is associated with significant mortality, urgent referral for haemodialysis should be considered (Wyatt et al., 2006).

### Tricyclic poisoning
Tricyclic anti-depressant medication is prescribed to relieve the symptoms of depressive illness and reduce the risk of suicide. Tricyclics are still widely prescribed for depression, despite the availability of newer selective serotonin-re-uptake inhibitors (SSRIs), which are associated with less morbidity and mortality

following overdose; tricyclics are less expensive than SSRIs and are considered by some to be more effective (Kerr et al., 2001). Tricyclic drugs most commonly involved in poisoning are dothiepin and amitriptyline, both of which have been found to be more toxic than other tricyclic medication (Henry et al., 1995).

Ingestion of 20 mg/kg is unlikely to produce toxicity although beyond this there is apparently little relationship between dose ingested and prognosis (Kerr et al., 2001).

### Side effects

Side effects include tachycardia, hypotension, widening of QRS complexes, cardiac arrhythmias, CNS depression, drowsiness, coma, convulsions and respiratory depression. The cardiotoxic effects occur within 6 h of ingestion; later complications are rare (Banahan & Schelkun, 1990).

### Specific treatment

Administration of activated charcoal to decontaminate the gut is indicated in patients who present within 1 h of ingesting >4 mg/kg, as long as the airway is safe and protected (Wyatt et al., 2006); continuous ECG monitoring to detect cardiac arrhythmias; cardiac arrhythmias should be treated by correcting hypoxia and acidosis: administer sodium bicarbonate 8.4% 50–100 ml IV (a further dose may be required) (Wyatt et al., 2006). Sodium bicarbonate can also help to correct hypotension and reverse widening of QRS complexes (Kerr et al., 2001). Anti-arrhythmic drugs should not be administered for cardiac arrhythmias as many interact with tricyclics and exacerbate the symptoms of poisoning, particular the cardiotoxic effects (Kerr et al., 2001). Cardiac monitoring should continue until the patient has had a normal reading for 12–24 h (Kerr et al., 2001).

### Opiate poisoning

Opiate poisoning is a major health problem in Western societies and its prevalence is increasing. Concomitant use of alcohol and/

or other drugs is associated with increased morbidity and mortality (Warner-Smith et al., 2001). It is most common among regular users of opium or heroin when it is accidentally taken in overdose or is combined with other drugs and/or alcohol to produce toxic side effects (Warner-Smith et al., 2001; Karbakhsh & Zandi, 2007). Potent opiates include heroin (diamorphine), morphine, fentanyl, buprenorphine and pethidine, and less potent compounds include codeine and tramadol.

*Side effects*
Side effects include pinpoint pupils, respiratory depression and bradypnoea, hypotension and altered consciousness or coma. Patients with a decreasing level of consciousness, bradypnoea and pinpoint pupils, where diagnosis is otherwise unclear (as the patient may present in coma or with a conscious level that precludes accurate history-taking), should be assumed to have taken opiates in overdose and provided with appropriate treatment. Patients without these clinical signs are unlikely to have taken opiates (Hoffman et al., 1991).

*Specific treatment*
Administer naloxone (narcan) 0.4 mg IV; repeated doses or an IV infusion may be required (Resuscitation Council, 2006). Intranasal naloxone is also clinically effective and has the advantage of not exposing staff to potential needlestick injury (Barton et al., 2005). Some patients may require tracheal intubation and ventilatory support.

**Barbituate poisoning**
Barbiturates, for example phenobarbitone, have been largely replaced in the treatment of anxiety and insomnia by benzodiazepines, mainly due to concerns about their toxicity in overdose. They can also cause dependency; addiction to these drugs remains a health concern (MedlinePlus, 2007). Barbituate poisoning is now uncommon, except among drug addicts (Wyatt et al., 2006).

Secondary to reduced prescription and improving critical care techniques mortality associated with barbiturate overdose has declined markedly with most remaining deaths being due to respiratory depression caused by long-acting barbiturates (Habal, 2006). Patients with delayed presentation, or those taking a large overdose, will need respiratory support and probably tracheal intubation.

*Side effects*
Side effects include sluggishness, poor co-ordination and unsteady gait, difficulty in thinking and slowness of speech, respiratory depression, drowsiness or coma.

*Specific investigations*
Investigations should include arterial blood gas analysis, and where resources are available plasma concentration of barbiturates may be of prognostic value.

*Specific treatment*
Decontamination of the gut with activated charcoal is indicated if the patient presents within an hour of ingestion but this should be undertaken with caution due to the risk of aspiration in a patient with a decreasing level of consciousness and poor respiratory effort (Greene & Lafferty, 2005). Tracheal intubation and activated charcoal admininstered via a naso-gastric tube may be required. As in overdose of aspirin and tricyclic antidepressant drugs alkalinisation of the urine by IV administration of sodium bicarbonate will enhance the elimination of longer-acting barbiturates (Greene & Lafferty, 2005). As there is no specific antidotal therapy for barbiturate overdose treatment is principally supportive.

**Benzodiazepine poisoning**
Benzodiazepines, for example diazepam, temazepam and nitrazepam, are used as sedative-hypnotic agents for the treatment of anxiety disorders, symptoms of alcohol withdrawal and insom-

nia, as well as during conscious sedation procedures and in pre-anaesthesia. Benzodiazepines are more common in overdose than barbiturates but their relative safety in overdose compared with barbiturates means that morbidity and mortality are of lesser significance. Death from isolated benzodiazepine overdose is rare and where death does occur it is often associated with the concomitant ingestion of other medication and/or alcohol (Mantooth, 2006). History-taking should therefore include inquiry about other medication and alcohol ingestion.

### Side effects
Side effects include dizziness and blurred vision, confusion, anxiety, agitation, drowsiness, unresponsiveness, coma, slurred speech, ataxia, hallucinations and amnesia, nystagmus, hypotonia and, rarely, respiratory depression and hypotension.

### Specific treatment
If only a benzodiazepine has been taken, gastric lavage and activated charcoal are not required; supportive treatment is all that is usually needed (Wyatt et al., 2006). Flumazenil is the specific antidote for a benzodiazepine but its use is associated with severe adverse side effects (Mantooth, 2006); for example, it can cause acute withdrawal symptoms in patients dependent on benzodiazepines and in combination with tricyclic anti-depressants it can cause seizures and cardiac arrest; therefore, it is only very occasionally used and only by an expert practitioner (Wyatt et al., 2006).

### Beta-blocker poisoning
Although no longer recommended for the primary treatment of hypertension (NICE, 2006), beta-blockers are still widely used for this purpose as well as for ischaemic heart disease secondary treatment.

### Side effects
Side effects include profound hypotension and cardiogenic shock (Wyatt et al., 2006), bradycardia, which may be marked and

resistant to atropine therapy (Slater, 2001), respiratory depression and coma.

*Specific investigations*
Investigations should include 12-lead ECG and blood glucose testing.

*Specific treatment*
Administration of activated charcoal to decontaminate the gut is indicated in patients who present within 1 h of ingesting; glucagon 5–10 mg IV is generally very effective at reversing the cardiovascular side effects; cardiac pacing may be required.

**Alcohol poisoning**
Alcohol poisoning is common and it can potentiate the CNS effects of other drugs. The widespread availability of alcohol and its relative inexpensiveness, along with a culture of binge drinking, mean that the incidence of alcohol poisoning is on the increase.

The relatively rapid absorption of alcohol in the gut makes the administration of activated charcoal of less therapeutic value than in other forms of overdose. In the absence of a specific antidote for alcohol, treatment is aimed at supporting the patient's vital functions. Alcohol can deplete hepatic reserves of glycogen, leading to hypoglycaemia.

In general a patient should only assumed to be drunk when all other causes of symptoms have been excluded and this may not be evident until the spontaneous restoration of normal activity as alcohol levels fall.

*Side effects*
Side effects include nausea and vomiting, decreased level of consciousness, coma and respiratory depression.

*Specific investigations*
Investigations should include blood glucose and blood alcohol levels.

*Specific treatment*
The airway may need to be secured as the patient's level of consciousness decreases and the risk of aspiration of stomach contents rises (Brick, 2005); severe respiratory depression may require assisted ventilation. Correct hypoglycaemia with IV glucose; look for other possible causes of altered conscious level including injuries (Wyatt et al., 2006). Patients with alcohol poisoning should therefore be closely observed and, where possible, a history should be taken from the patient, family or friends to try to establish medical history and whether there are any concomitant injuries.

**Ecstasy**
Ecstasy is an amphetamine derivative, which is used as a stimulant.

*Side effects*
Side effects include tachycardia, agitation, sweating, hypertension followed by hypotension, pyrexia; in severe cases coma, heat stroke, seizures, cardiac arrhythmia; metabolic acidosis, hyperkalaemia, hypoglycaemia and hyponatraemia can occur (Wyatt et al., 2006). Rhabdomyolitis may also occur.

*Specific investigations*
Investigations should include arterial blood gas analysis, urea and electrolyes, blood glucose CK, liver function tests and 12-lead ECG.

*Specific treatment*
Administration of activated charcoal to decontaminate the gut is indicated in patients who present within 1 h of ingesting; supportive treatment, if the rectal temperature is above 40°C dantrolene 1 mg/kg IV should be administered; further doses may be required (Wyatt et al., 2006). Correct acidosis with sodium bicarbinate and correct hypoglycaemia.

## SUMMARY

Overdose of medication causes a variety of toxic effects and this may be complicated by patients taking a mixture of different drugs and sometimes ingesting these with alcohol. Patients who delay presentation may also present a variety of clinical challenges. Where specific antidotes for poisoning are available, then these should be administered providing the patient has presented in appropriate time after ingestion. Expert advice should always be sought.

All patients who have taken an overdose in an attempt to harm themselves should have an estimate of suicidal intent made and there are clinical tools to aid this process. The prevention of further self-harm is as important as the treatment of the consequences.

## REFERENCES

Arbuthnot, L & Gillespie, M (2005) Self-harm: reviewing psychological assessment in emergency departments. *Emergency Nurse* **12**(10), 20–4

Banahan, B & Schelkun, P (1990) Tricyclic antidepressant overdosage: conservative management in a community hospital with cost-saving implications. *Journal of Emergency Medicine* **8**, 451–4

Barton, E, Colwell, C, Wolfe, T, Fosnocht, D, Gravitz, C, Bryan, T, et al. (2005) Efficacy of intranasal naloxone as a needleless alternative for treatment of opioid overdose in the prehospital setting. *Journal of Emergency Medicine* **29**(3), 265–71

BMJ Clinical Evidence (2006) Paracetamol (acetaminophen) poisoning. BMJ Publishing, London. http://clinicalevidence.bmj.com/ceweb/conditions/pos/2101/2101_references.jsp (accessed 4 April 2007)

Brick, J (2005) *Alcohol Overdose*. New Brunswick Center of Alcohol Studies, New Brunswick, NJ. http://alcoholstudies.rutgers.edu/onlinefacts/od.html (accessed 4 April 2007)

Department of Health (1999) *National Service Framework for Mental Health*. Department of Health, London

Farley, A, Hendry, C & Napier, P (2005) Paracetamol poisoning: Physiological aspects and management strategies. *Nursing Standard* **19**(38), 58–64

Farmer, C & Bethel, J (2006) Evaluating suicidal intent in emergency care settings. *Emergency Nurse* **14**(7), 20–4

Galea, S, Ahern, J, Vlahov, D, Coffin, P, Fuller, C, Leon, A & Tardiff, K (2003) Income distribution and risk of fatal drug overdose in New York City neighbourhoods. *Drug and Alcohol Dependence* **70**, 139–48

Goldsack, N, Howell, D, Marshall, R & Montgomery, H (1999) Emergency! *British Medical Journal*. www.studentbmj.com/back_issues/0699/data/0699ed1.htm (accessed 31 March 2007)

Greene, T & Lafferty, K (2005) *Barbiturate Toxicity*. e-medicine. com. www.emedicine.com/emerg/topic52.htm (accessed 4 April 2007)

Gunnell, D, Ho, D & Murray, V (2004) Medical management of deliberate drug overdose: A neglected area for suicide prevention? *Emergency Medical Journal* **21**, 35–8

Habal, R (2006) *Toxicity, Barbiturates*. e-medicine.com. www.emedicine.com/med/topic207.htm (accessed 4 April 2007)

Hartley, V (2002) Paracetamol overdose. *Emergency Nurse* **10**(5), 17–24

Hawton, K, Townsend, E, Deeks, J, Appleby, L, Gunnell, D, Bennewith, O & Cooper, J (2001) Effects of legislation restricting pack sizes of paracetamol and salicylate on self poisoning in the UK: before and after study. *British Medical Journal* **322**, 1203–7

Henry, J, Alexander, C & Sener, E (1995) Relative mortality from overdose of antidepressants. *British Medical Journal* **310**, 221–4

Hockberger, R & Rothstein, R (1988) Assessment of suicide potential by nonpsychiatrists using the sad persons score. *Journal of Emergency Medicine* **6**, 99–107

Hoffman, J, Schriger, D & Luo, J (1991) The empiric use of naloxone in patients with altered mental status: a reappraisal. *Annals of Emergency Medicine* **20**(3), 246–52

Horrocks, J (2002) Self-poisoning and self-injury in adults. *Clinical Medicine* **2**(6), 509–12

Hume, M & Platt, S (2007) Appropriate interventions for the prevention and management of self-harm: a qualitative exploration of service-users' views. *BMC Public Health*. www.pubmedcentral.nih.gov/picrender.fcgi?artid=1790886&blobtype=pdf (accessed 31 March 2007)

Kamanyire, R (2002) Aspirin overdose. *Emergency Nurse* **10**(4), 17–22

Kapur, N, House, A, Creed, F, Feldman, E, Friedman, T & Guthrie, E (1998) Management of deliberate self-poisoning in adults in four teaching hospitals: descriptive study. *British Medical Journal* **316**, 831–2

Kapur, N, House, A, Dodgson, K, May, C, Marshall, S, Tomenson, B & Creed, F (2002) Management and costs of deliberate self-poisoning in the general hospital: a multi-centre study. *Journal of Mental Health* **11**(2), 223–30

Karbakhsh, M & Zandi, N (2007) Acute opiate overdose in Tehran: the forgotten role of opium. *Addictive Behaviours* **32**(9), 1835–42

Kerr, G, McGuffie, A & Wilkie, S (2001) Tricyclic antidepressant overdose: a review. *Emergency Medical Journal* **18**, 236–41

Laye-Gindhu, A & Schonert-Reichl, K (2005) Nonsuicidal self-harm among community adolescents: understanding the 'whats' and 'whys' of self-harm. *Journal of Youth and Adolescence* **34**(5), 447–57

Mackay, N & Barrowclough, C (2005) Accident and emergency staff's perceptions of deliberate self-harm: attributions, emotions and willingness to help. *British Journal of Clinical Psychology* **44**(2), 255–67

Mantooth, R (2006) *Toxicity, Benzodiazepines*. e-medicine.com. www.emedicine.com/EMERG/topic58 (accessed 4 April 2007)

Mayo Foundation for Medical Health and Research (2006) *Self injury/cutting*. RevolutionHealth. www.revolutionhealth.com/healthy-living/parenting/ages-stages/high-school/issues/cutting-self-injury (accessed 31 March 2007)

McAllister, M, Creedy, D, Moyle, W & Farrugia, C (2002) Nurses' attitudes towards clients who self-harm. *Journal of Advanced Nursing* **40**(5), 578–86

Medicines and Healthcare Products Regulatory Agency (2005) *Salicylates and Aspirin Overdose*. MHRA, London. www.mhra. gov.uk/home/idcplg?IdcService=SS_GET_PAGE&nodeId= 792 (accessed 1 April 2007)

MedlinePlus (2007) *Barbiturate Intoxication and Overdose*. National Institutes of Health and US National Library of Medicine. www.nlm.nih.gov/medlineplus/ency/article/000951. htm#Alternative%20Names (accessed 4 April 2007)

NICE (2004) *Self Harm: the Short-term Physical and Psychological Management and Secondary Prevention of Self Harm in Primary and Secondary Care*. NICE, London. http://guidance.nice.org.uk/ CG16/?c=91523 (accessed 31 March 2007)

NICE (2006) *Hypertension: Management of Hypertension in Adults in Primary Care*. NICE, London. http://guidance.nice.org.uk/ CG34 (accessed 4 April 2007)

Office for National Statistics (2005) Mortality from suicide and drug-related poisoning by day of the week in England and Wales 1993–2002. *Health Statistics Quarterly* (27). www.statis-tics.gov.uk/downloads/theme_health/HSQ27_superseded. pdf (accessed 31 March 2007)

Office for National Statistics (2007) Latest UK suicide figures released. *Health Statistics Quarterly* (33). www.statistics. gov.uk/downloads/theme_health/hsq33web.pdf (accessed 31 March 2007)

Owens, D, Horrocks, J & House, A, (2002) Fatal and non-fatal repetition of self-harm: systematic review. *British Journal of Psy-chiatry* **181**, 193–9

Parker, D (1990) Safety of late acetylcysteine treatment in paracetamol poisoning. *Human and Experimental Toxicology* **9**, 25–7

Preti, A, Miotto, P & De Coppi, M (2002) Deaths by unintentional illicit drug overdose in Italy, 1984–2000. *Drug and Alcohol Dependence* **66**, 275–82

Resuscitation Council UK (2006) *Advanced Life Support Provider Manual, 5th edn*. Resuscitation Council UK, London.

Royal College of Psychiatrists (1994) *The General Hospital Management of Adult Deliberate Self-Harm: A Consensus Statement on Standards for Service Provision*. Council Report Number 32. Royal College of Psychiatrists, London

Samaritans (2005) *Self-harm and Suicide*. Samaritans, London. www.samaritans.org.uk/know/information/information-sheets/selfharm/selfharm_sheet.shtm#overview (accessed 31 March 2007)

Schmidt, L & Dalhoff, K (2002) Concomitant overdosing of other drugs in patients with paracetamol poisoning. *British Journal of Clinical Pharmacology* **53**, 535–41

Singleton, N, Pendry, E, Taylor, C, Farrell, M & Marsden, J (2003) *Drug-related Mortality Among Newly Released Offenders*. Home Office Research Development and Statistics Directorate, London. www.homeoffice.gov.uk/rds/pdfs2/r187.pdf (accessed 31 March 2007)

Slater, T (2001) A 39 year old man with an overdose of β–blockers. *Journal of Emergency Nursing* **27**, 323–6

Warner-Smith, M, Darke, S, Lynskey, M & Hall, W (2001) Heroin overdose: causes and consequences. *Addiction* **96**, 1113–25

World Health Organization (2003) *Suicide Rates (per 100,000), by Country, Year, and Gender*. World Health Organization, Geneva. www.who.int/mental_health/prevention/suicide/suiciderates/en/ (accessed 31 March 2007)

Wyatt, J, Illingworth, R, Graham, C, Clancy, M & Robertson, C (2006) *Oxford Handbook of Emergency Medicine*, 3rd edn. Oxford University Press, Oxford

# Critical Care Outreach Service

# 11

Kate Deacon

## INTRODUCTION

Critical care outreach services (CCOSs) have been developed in England following recommendations made in *Critical to Success* (Audit Commission, 1999) and *Comprehensive Critical Care – a Review of Adult Critical Care Services* (Department of Health, 2000). They have been established in accordance with the philosophy of 'intensive care without walls' as one aspect of the critical care service (Gwinnutt, 2006). All Acute Trusts should have this service available 24 h a day, 7 days a week (National Confidential Enquiry into Patient Outcome and Death (NCEPOD, 2005).

Despite widespread acceptance and an intuitive belief of the benefit of CCOSs, there is a lack of evidence to support their use, there are national variations in their availability and there is no consensus about the ideal composition (Holder & Cuthbertson, 2005)

The aim of this chapter is to allow the reader to understand the role of the CCOS.

## LEARNING OUTCOMES

By the end of the chapter the reader will be able to:

❏ discuss the background to critical care outreach services (CCOSs),
❏ state the objectives of CCOSs,
❏ demonstrate an awareness of how outreach services have developed and the issues involved in their implementation,
❏ describe the use track and trigger systems and the importance of physiological observations.

## BACKGROUND TO CRITICAL CARE OUTREACH SERVICES (CCOSS)

### Comprehensive Critical Care

The report *Comprehensive Critical Care* (Department of Health, 2000) provides a framework for the future organisation and delivery of adult critical care services in England. The report acknowledged that critical care service provision had developed over the years in a haphazard and unplanned manner with a significant amount of variation between NHS Trusts. The aim of the report was to ensure there was consistency in the standard of care for patients who were either critically ill, or crucially, at risk of becoming so, whether in the intensive care unit (ICU)/high-dependency unit (HDU) or in a ward environment.

### 'Intensive care without walls'

The report's philosophy of intensive care without walls proposed a move away from critical care being a service just received by patients who were on an ICU or HDU, to a service that was focused on how unwell the patient was regardless of geographical location.

### Classification of patients

The report proposed a system for classifying patients according to the level of care required (Box 11.1). Levels ranged from 0, representing a patient whose needs could be met on a normal acute hospital ward, to level 3, which represented patients requiring the highest level of support normally cared for in an ICU. This was the report's key recommendation upon which all other recommendations were based (Department of Health, 2000).

### Proposal for CCOS

The move to classify patients according to level of need was the basis of a number of proposals that aimed to bring about a critical care service that was integrated into the hospital-wide bed management. There were four key proposals for the content of the

---

**Box 11.1 Levels of care classification**

Level 0   Patients whose needs can be met through normal ward care in an acute hospital.

Level 1   Patients at risk of their condition deteriorating, or those recently relocated from higher levels of care, whose needs can be met on an acute ward with additional advice and support from the critical care team.

Level 2   Patients requiring more detailed observation or intervention including support for a single failing organ system or post-operative care and those 'stepping down' from higher levels of care.

Level 3   Patients requiring advanced respiratory support alone or basic respiratory support together with support of at least two organ systems. This level includes all complex patients requiring support for multi-organ failure.

Source: Department of Health (2000).

---

critical care service, the first of which was the establishment of CCOS to support the care of level 1 patients on general wards. This classification system officially recognised the existence of patients on the wards whose condition deteriorates such that they need a level of care beyond the normal level of care for that area.

The report acknowledged that a significant number of patients deteriorate on wards and receive sub-optimal care; this sub-optimal care could be through a combination of failure to detect deterioration and failure to respond effectively, the consequences of which had serious effects on patient outcome (Schein et al., 1990; McQuillan et al., 1998). CCOSs were one of the key proposals to try and tackle this problem.

The establishing of CCOSs was one of a large number of proposals made for comprehensive critical care as part of an overall framework to modernise and standardise critical care services in

England. Whereas some of its recommendations were meant for immediate implementation, the timescale proposed for CCOSs, along with several other recommendations was 3–5 years (Department of Health, 2000).

## OBJECTIVES OF THE CCOS

The objectives of CCOSs are to:

- avert ICU admissions by identifying patients who are deteriorating and either helping to prevent admission or ensuring that admission to a critical care bed happens in a timely manner to ensure best outcome;
- enable ICU discharges by supporting both the continuing recovery of discharged patients on wards and after discharge from hospital;
- share critical care skills with staff in wards and the community, ensuring enhancement of training opportunities and skills practice and using information gathered from the ward and community to improve critical care services for patients and relatives.

(Department of Health, 2000)

## IMPLEMENTATION AND DEVELOPMENT OF CCOS

All Acute Trusts should have a formal CCOS that is available 24 h a day, 7 days a week (NCEPOD, 2005). The composition of this service will vary from hospital to hospital but it should comprise individuals with the skills and ability to recognise and manage the problems of critical illness (NCEPOD, 2005). Outreach services should not replace the role of traditional medical teams in the care of inpatients, but should be seen as complementary (NCEPOD, 2005).

However, many outreach services are often not available on a 24-h basis (NCEPOD, 2005). Some only provide cover for selected patients, for example post-operative surgery (NCEPOD, 2005). Forty-four per cent of hospitals do not even provide an outreach service (NCEPOD, 2005), although McDonnell et al. (2008) found that 72.8% of hospitals now do.

Current recommendations state that CCOSs should be available 24 h a day, 7 days a week (Intensive Care Society, 2002; Department of Health, 2005; NICE Short Clinical Guidelines Technical Team, 2007); however, only 33.8% offered 24-h support. For some of these services the cover that was available for 24 h consisted of telephone support; those services that offered clinical support on the ward 24 h a day was just 14.5%.

The professional make-up of the CCOS may be entirely nursing or multi-professional. Multi-professional CCOSs by their very nature will have an advantage when communicating with different disciplines across hospital environments. The majority of CCOSs that have shown measurable benefits have been multi-professional (Cutler & Robson, 2006). There has been shown to be variety in the amount of medical input into CCOSs and most services are nurse-led; 71.1% of services have no medical input at all (McDonnell et al., 2008).

The approach of the CCOS will vary depending on how much the emphasis of the service is on education and advice and how much it is on direct intervention to patient management. Current recommendations of a multi-professional service provided 24 h a day, 7 days a week, responding to so-called track and trigger referrals (see below), is firmly of the interventionist approach. This is not surprising or unreasonable given concerns over sub-optimal care of level 1 patients and the serious consequences this can have. However, as noted by Cutler and Robson (2006) these services are very expensive to implement and will only directly influence the care of patients it has contact with. Educationalist approaches will aim to educate the staff caring for patients who are potentially at risk of critical illness and in this way may influence the care of a larger number of patients. Therefore it would seem that any CCOS should combine both aspects. This is in line with recommendations that CCOS should be there to support, enable and work with ward staff, not to diminish them and take over responsibility (Intensive Care Society, 2002; Department of Health, 2005). However, resource constraints have been shown to be a factor in developing services for some trusts (McDonnell et al., 2008).

Alternatives to the CCOS include medical emergency teams (MET) and patient at-risk teams (PART). The MET developed in Australia in the early 1990s. The team was predominantly medical and replaced the cardiac arrest team; it aimed to intervene in the care of patients before they reached the point of cardiac arrest to try to and improve outcome, thus recognising that most patients will display physiological deterioration for several hours before cardiac arrest (Cutler & Robson, 2006). PARTs are separate from cardiac arrest teams and tend to be nurse-led. Unlike CCOSs and PARTs, METs are not an approach commonly used in the UK (NICE Short Clinical Guidelines Technical Team, 2007).

## 'TRACK AND TRIGGER' SYSTEMS

'Track and trigger' systems use sets of physiological observations to track the patient's clinical state; when a pre-set parameter is reached a defined response is triggered. Different types of track and trigger system exist, some using multiple parameters and some using just one. The MET uses a single-parameter system; satisfying any one of a specified list of criteria can trigger a call to the MET. The PART uses a multiple parameter system where a set number of criteria need to be met from a specified list to trigger a call.

CCOSs are triggered by a variety of systems, the most common in the UK being the modified early warning score (MEWS) (NCEPOD, 2005). This is an aggregate system where weighted scores are assigned to values for different physiological criteria; these scores are then totalled and the required response depends on the score. Response criteria may be listed or in the form of an algorithm. The main advantages of early warning score systems are:

- simplicity: only the basic monitoring equipment is required (usually readily available on acute wards);

- reproducibility between different observers;
- applicability to multi-professional team;
- minimal staff training required.

(Gwinnutt, 2006)

In recent clinical guidance relating to the acutely ill hospital patient the NICE Short Clinical Guidelines Technical Team (2007) reviewed available evidence relating to track and trigger systems being used internationally. Although the evidence was able to suggest some pros and cons of different systems it was felt that there was not sufficient evidence to recommend one particular system over another. The NICE Short Clinical Guidelines Technical Team (2007) recommends that *all* adult patients in acute hospital settings should be monitored with a track and trigger system but the choice of which particular system to use should be decided at a local level. However, it is recommended that the track and trigger systems used should have either multiple-parameter or aggregate scoring systems as these allow for a graded response, which is recommended (NICE Short Clinical Guidelines Technical Team, 2007).

Recommendations as to how often the physiological observations making up these scores should be performed and what these should consist of (as a minimum) have also been made. The recommendations apply to 'adult patients in acute hospital settings including patients in the emergency department for whom a clinical decision to admit has been made' (NICE Short Clinical Guidelines Technical Team, 2007: p.8). Recommendations are summarised in Box 11.2.

All of the recommendations above highlight the importance of basic assessment of physiological observations and the fact they are fundamental to providing adequate care. The degrees of abnormality detected in physiological observations have been shown to have a direct relationship to mortality rates (Goldhill et al., 2005; NCEPOD, 2005). It could be expected that as basic observations can give such an important insight into a patient's condition that they would be rigorously completed and acted upon. However,

**Box 11.2 Summary of NICE Short Clinical Guidelines Technical Team (2007) recommendations for physiological observations**

Observations should be taken at the time of admission initial assessment.

A clear written plan should be made recording which observations are to be recorded and how often.

Observations should be recorded and acted upon by staff who have been trained to undertake them and understand their relevance.

Physiological track and trigger systems should be used to monitor all patients.

Physiological observations should be monitored at least every 12 h unless a decision has been made to decrease this at a senior level.

Frequency of monitoring should increase if abnormal physiology is detected as outlined in the graded response strategy.

The following should form routine monitoring: heart rate, respiratory rate, systolic blood pressure, level of consciousness, $SaO_2$ and temperature (as a minimum).

practice has not reflected this. Evidence shows consistently that patients who become acutely unwell on hospital wards receive sub-optimal care because of delays in detecting and appropriately responding to deterioration, which have contributed to morbidity and mortality (McQuillan et al., 1998; NCEPOD, 2005).

The National Confidential Enquiry into Patient Outcome and Death (NCEPOD, 2005) found that despite respiratory rate being the physiological observation most sensitive to detecting deterioration it was the observation least often performed. A specific recommendation was made in their report that the importance of respiratory rate should be highlighted and that respiratory rate should be recorded whenever other observations are being made (NCEPOD, 2005).

The monitoring of physiological observations, however, is only the first step in a chain of events that needs to happen for the acutely ill patient to receive appropriate care. The staff member recording the observations needs to understand the implications of what they are monitoring so they know whether further action is necessary. If further action is deemed necessary then medical review of patients needs to be timely when requested by ward staff and finally when the medical team reviews the patient's condition they need to instigate appropriate action (including contacting their seniors where necessary), again in a timely manner. Evidence regarding sub-optimal care of acutely ill ward patients has found shortcomings at all stages of this chain (NCEPOD, 2005).

In view of these issues track and trigger tools aim to offer an objective guide for ward staff as to when they need to be taking further action in response to patient observations, thus support-ing them in these decisions. Some patients, however, will be able to physiologically compensate as they become critically ill and their deterioration may not show in observations until a later stage than may be expected (Intensive Care Society, 2003). It is therefore widely agreed that intuition that a patient is not quite right and is causing ward staff concern should remain a legiti-mate reason for referral to CCOS in the absence of a triggering score (Intensive Care Society, 2003; NICE Short Clinical Guide-lines Technical Team, 2007).

As mentioned above the MEWS is an example of an aggregate scoring track and trigger system and is used widely in the UK (NICE Short Clinical Guidelines Technical Team, 2007). Table 11.1 shows an example of the MEWS system.

Following recording of a set of physiological observations a score is calculated and recorded using a table such as the example in Table 11.1. A graded set of response criteria can then be referred to as discussed above to decide what further action is needed. Implementation of a track and trigger scoring system can be considered by applying the MEWS system to the case study in Box 11.3. To establish whether further action would be required for Mrs B a MEWS score of 3 or over will be taken as a trigger for action.

**Table 11.1** MEWS scoring system

| | Points | | | | | | |
|---|---|---|---|---|---|---|---|
| | 3 | 2 | 1 | 0 | 1 | 2 | 3 |
| Systolic blood pressure (mmHg) | <70 | 71–80 | 81–100 | 101–199 | | ≥200 | |
| Heart rate (beats/min) | | <40 | 41–50 | 51–100 | 101–110 | 111–129 | >130 |
| Respiratory rate (breaths/min) | | <9 | | 9–14 | 15–20 | 21–29 | >30 |
| Temperature (°C) | | <35 | | 35–38.4 | | >38.5 | |
| Neurological score (AVPU) | | | | **A**lert | Reacting to **v**oice | Reacting to **p**ain | **U**nresponsive |

From Subbe et al. (2003).

---

**Box 11.3 Case study of Mrs B**

Mrs B is 58-year-old lady who was admitted to the ward the previous evening with a history of diarrhoea and vomiting. She has had a restless night complaining of abdominal discomfort and thirst. She has been given analgesia and an IV infusion of 1 litre of 0.9% NaCl was commenced at 22:00 the previous evening to run over 12 h. At 10:00 her observations are taken and found to be as follows.

Heart rate: 118 beats/min
Respiratory rate: 34 breaths/min
Blood pressure: 110/55 mmHg
Temperature: 38°C
SaO$_2$: 94%
Neurological status: alert

What would be Mrs B's MEWS score based on these observations?
    What else would you want to know from the information given above?

Calculating Mrs B's MEWS score from the available data, a score of 5 would be obtained:

- heart rate: 118 beats/min = 2 points,
- respiratory rate: 34 breaths/min = 3 points,
- systolic blood pressure: 110 mmHg = 0 points,
- temperature: 38°C = 0 points,
- $SaO_2$: 94% = not on scoring tool,
- neurological status: alert = 0 points.

A score of 5 would trigger a response according to an agreed criteria/algorithm. If the respiratory rate had not been counted, the MEWS score would have fallen from 5 to 2 and may have failed to trigger a response. This is a crucial point as respiratory rate is often omitted from observation rounds (NCEPOD, 2005). Respiratory rate should always be recorded.

From the other information, Mrs B's fluid status is cause for concern, as she has been admitted with diarrhoea and was complaining of thirst overnight. A check would need to be made to ensure that an accurate fluid-balance chart has been maintained, and what her current fluid balance is. An assessment of Mrs B's pain would need to be made to ascertain whether the analgesia has been effective; the type and severity of the pain should be documented. This information can then be handed over to the medical team.

The NICE Short Clinical Guidelines Technical Team (2007) guidelines suggest that beyond the monitoring of the minimum physiological observations consideration should also be given to monitoring biochemistry, hourly urine and pain. These investigations would all be appropriate in the case of Mrs B.

At a local level variations exist as to the scoring system that is used (even within one system such as the MEWS minor variations in parameters can be seen), and the formats for guiding staff as to the course of action that needs to be taken. However, what is fundamentally important in practice in every acute hospital is that an agreed system exists which staff use and understand and that works to optimise the care given to acutely ill ward patients.

SUMMARY

Following the publication of *Comprehensive Critical Care* (Department of Health, 2000) CCOSs have been widely developed, although there is considerable variety as to how these services are implemented. Track and trigger systems are employed to identify patients of concern and for whom input of the CCOS may be required. A number of different systems exist but all use basic physiological observations. Recent clinical guidance from the NICE Short Clinical Guidelines Technical Team (2007) recommends that whichever system is used the core observations to be measured should be: heart rate, respiratory rate, systolic blood pressure, conscious level, $SaO_2$ and temperature. Issues that impact the implementation and running of CCOSs include hours of cover, skill mix, funding and education. A body of research relating to CCOS is starting to develop, but at present a conclusive evidence base which can tell us the most effective methods for identifying and responding to acutely ill patients is still awaited. What remains clear is that some acutely unwell patients continue to be at risk of receiving suboptimal care with potentially severe or even life-threatening consequences. Therefore, continued work aiming to optimise the care for the acutely unwell patient is vital.

REFERENCES

Audit Commission (1999) *Critical to Success: The Place of Efficient and Effective Critical Care Services within the Acute Hospital.* Audit Commission: London. www.auditcommission.gov.uk/ publications/pdf/nrccare.pdf (accessed 21 January 2008)

Cutler, L & Robson, W (eds) (2006) *Critical Care Outreach.* John Wiley & Sons, Chichester

Department of Health (2000) *Comprehensive Critical Care – a Review of Adult Critical Care Services.* Department of Health, London

Department of Health (2005) *Quality Critical Care – Beyond Comprehensive Critical Care.* Department of Health, London

Goldhill, DR, McNarry, AF, Mandershoot, G & McGinley, A (2005) A physiologically based early warning score for ward patients: the association between score and outcome. *Anaesthesia* **60**, 547–53

Gwinnutt, C (2006) *Clinical Anaesthesia*, 2nd edn. Blackwell Publishing, Oxford

Holder, P & Cuthbertson, BH (2005) Critical care outwith the intensive care unit. *Journal of the Royal College of Physicians* **5**(5), 449–51

Intensive Care Society (2002) *Guidelines for the Introduction of Outreach Services*. Intensive Care Society, London

Intensive Care Society (2003) *The National Outreach Report*. Department of Health and Modernisation Agency, London. www.dh.gov.uk/prod_consum_dh/groups/dh_digitalassets/@dh/@en/documents/digitalasset/dh_4063500.pdf (accessed 21 January 2008)

McDonnell, A, Esmonde, L, Morgan, R, Brown, R, Bray, K, Parry, G, et al. (2008) The provision of critical care outreach services in England: findings from a national survey. *Journal of Critical Care* (in press)

McQuillan, P, Pilkington, S, Allan, A & Taylor, B, et al. (1998) Confidential enquiry into quality of care before admission to intensive care. *British Medical Journal* **316**(7148), 1853–8

National Confidential Enquiry into Patient Outcome and Death (2005) *An Acute Problem?* National Confidential Enquiry into Patient Outcome and Death, London

NICE Short Clinical Guidelines Technical Team (2007) *Acutely Ill Patients in Hospital – Recognition of and Response to Acute Illness in Adults in Hospital*. NICE, London

Schein, RM, Hazday, N, Pena, M, Ruben, BH & Sprung, CL (1990) Clinical antecedents to in-hospital cardiopulmonary arrest. *Chest* **98**(6), 1388–92

Subbe, CP, Davies, RG, Williams, E, Rutherford, P & Gemmell, L (2003) Effect of introducing the Modified Early Warning score on clinical outcomes, cardio-pulmonary arrests and intensive care utilisation in acute medical admissions. *Anaesthesia* **58**, 797–802

# 12 | Ethical and Legal Issues

Fiona Foxall

## INTRODUCTION

All nurses working in the acute care setting will inevitably encounter the death of some of their patients. Death is the outcome of a process of dying that may be expected, unexpected, sudden or protracted. Whichever the case, the legal and ethical issues relating to end-of-life circumstances can evoke anxiety in nurses caring for such patients.

The aim of this chapter is to provide an overview of the ethical and legal issues frequently encountered in acute care settings related to critical illness and death.

## LEARNING OUTCOMES

At the end of the chapter the reader will be able to:

❏ outline the ethical theories and principles that guide health-care practice,
❏ discuss Do Not Attempt Resuscitation orders and advance directives,
❏ briefly outline the Mental Capacity Act 2005,
❏ discuss the ethics of withdrawal of active treatment,
❏ discuss the sanctity of life doctrine,
❏ outline the care objectives of palliative care in the acute setting.

## ETHICAL THEORIES AND PRINCIPLES THAT GUIDE HEALTHCARE PRACTICE

### Ethical theories

There are two major ethical theories which guide healthcare practice:

- **deontology** (duty-based theory), the basic tenet of which is, 'I must always carry out my duty';
- **utilitarianism** (consequence-based theory), which asserts that an action is right if it produces the greatest benefit for the greatest number of people.

Often, carrying out your duty will produce the best consequences but unfortunately this is not always the case.

### Ethical principles

There are four guiding ethical principles which should also be used in the decision-making process.

- **Nonmaleficence** (*primum non nocere*): first and above all, do no harm.
- **Beneficence**: do good, promote good, remove evil or harm.
- **Respect for autonomy**: taking into account and acting on the patient's wishes.
- **Justice**: fairness, entitlement or right.

(Beauchamp & Childress, 2001)

### Decision-making process

These theories and principles can aid in decision-making by asking six simple questions.

- What is my duty in this particular circumstance?
- By carrying out my duty, will my actions produce the best available consequences for all concerned?
- Will my actions harm anyone, particularly the patient?
- Am I going to do or promote good for those concerned?
- Am I respecting the patient's wishes?
- Are my actions fair?

This may over-simplify the decision-making process but provides a useful guide. *The Code of Professional Conduct* for nurses, midwives and health visitors (Nursing and Midwifery Council, 2008) takes these issues into account; so working within the confines of this Code will ensure that you act not only within the law but also in an ethical manner.

## DO NOT ATTEMPT RESUSCITATION ORDERS AND ADVANCE DIRECTIVES

### Do not attempt resuscitation orders

Cardiopulmonary resuscitation (CPR) is a procedure that is used to attempt to restore cardiac and/or respiratory function to individuals who have sustained a cardiac and/or respiratory arrest. Do Not Attempt Resuscitation (DNAR) is a medical order to withhold CPR in patients for whom resuscitation is futile or in patients who have mental capacity who have refused CPR.

Use of CPR gives the ability to reverse premature death. It can also prolong terminal illness, increase discomfort and consume enormous resources (Ewanchuck & Brindley, 2006). Only 10–20% of all those in whom CPR is attempted in acute general hospitals will live to be discharged (Bowker & Stewart, 1999). It is therefore clear that CPR is often futile and where possible medical staff will consider a DNAR order.

The concept of medical futility is important here and refers to interventions that are unlikely to produce any significant benefit for the patient. This can be in terms of either the likelihood that an intervention will benefit the patient or, if there is any benefit, the quality of that benefit. A treatment that merely produces a physiological effect on a patient's body does not necessarily confer any benefit that the patient can appreciate. The question is, does the intervention have any reasonable prospect of helping the patient (Jecker, 2000)?

Wherever possible a DNAR order should be made by all those involved in the patient's care, the patient's significant others and, most importantly, where the patient has the capacity to make

> **Box 12.1 When to consider a DNAR order**
>
> A decision that a patient should not be resuscitated should only take place where:
>
> 1 a mentally competent patient has refused treatment.
> 2 a valid living will covering such circumstances has been made by the patient.
> 3 effective CPR is unlikely to be successful.
> 4 successful CPR is likely to be followed by a length and quality of life that would not be in the best interests of the patient to sustain.
>
> Source: Dimond (2005).

decisions, the patient him- or herself. A DNAR order can be instigated under the conditions outlined in Box 12.1.

### Advance directives

Advance directives (also referred to as living wills, advance statements or advance refusals) are usually written directives from individuals who have mental capacity to healthcare professionals regarding treatment that should be provided or forgone in specific circumstances, during periods of incapacity (Beauchamp & Childress, 2001). However, an advance directive does not have to be written to be valid. If a patient makes a verbal advance statement that they do not wish to have a particular form of treatment should they become incapacitated, this must be respected. However, it must be ascertained that the advance directive is valid and this needs to be documented in the patient's medical and nursing notes.

A person is deemed to have capacity when they are able to make rational decisions based on appropriate information so that when cognitive impairment occurs, perhaps as a result of acute illness, it would be inappropriate for the person to write an advance directive at that time.

The trigger for using an advance directive is typically the occurrence of an acute clinical event in a patient with an enduring or degenerative condition that has already compromised quality of life as judged by the patient whilst he/she has capacity and does not wish their life to be protracted by artificial means.

Advance directives are rooted in respect for autonomy (Beauchamp & Childress, 2001), which is one of the foremost ethical principles. Western society places great importance on a person's right to self-determination even when he or she is unable to participate in decision-making due to incapacity (Bosek & Savage, 2007). As adult patients who have capacity have a right to refuse medical treatment, an advance directive is a way of prolonging autonomy. However, an advance directive cannot request treatment that is not in the best interests of the patient.

The legality of an advance directive is recognised at common law (i.e. judge-made law), as there is no Act of Parliament setting out the law. If the advance directive is signed and witnessed and the doctor believes this document to represent the wishes of the patient, the doctor can rely on its provisions as a defence if any actions are to be brought for their failure to treat the patient (Dimond, 2005).

### How DNAR orders and advance directives affect acute care

The major issues to consider here are autonomy and mental capacity. To consider how the concepts of DNAR and advance directives affect care in view of these issues, a series of case studies will be considered (see Boxes 12.2–12.5).

Autonomy addresses personal freedom and self-determination; that is, the right to choose what will happen to one's own person (within social and legal constraints). The legal doctrine of informed consent is a direct reflection of this principle. Autonomy involves healthcare deliverers' respect for patients' rights to make decisions affecting care and treatment, even if the healthcare deliverers do not agree with the decisions made (Wacker Guido, 2006).

---

**Box 12.2 Case study 1: autonomy**

Katie is a 38-year-old lady who has been admitted to undergo bilateral mastectomy for breast cancer. It is 1 hr before she is due to go for surgery and she states that she is now unwilling to have the surgery and wishes to go home. She says that she does not want any treatment other than painkillers and she is aware that as a result of this she will die. However, she would rather die than have treatment and live with no breasts.

Breast reconstruction has been discussed with her but she is now adamant that she does not want the surgery or any other treatment. Her husband and 14-year-old daughter are extremely upset and are insisting that she is forced to have the procedure.

What is the position of healthcare professionals in these circumstances?

---

Clearly, Katie (Case study 1, Box 12.2) has made an autonomous decision and her decision should be respected. The healthcare professionals caring for Katie should ensure she has all the appropriate information to ensure the decisions she makes are fully informed but her refusal should be accepted on that basis. Her family should be treated compassionately and given all information that Katie is happy for them to receive but no competent patient can be treated without informed consent, as this would constitute assault and battery. Katie has not given consent to treatment and her refusal constitutes an advance directive, albeit in an oral form.

Clearly, in view of the seriousness of his condition and because of his physical deterioration, it is unlikely that Frank (Case study 2, Box 12.3) would be able to make a sound judgement as he is mentally incapacitated by his condition. However, relatives have no right in law to refuse consent to any life-saving treatment required by the patient. The only criterion, in these circumstances, that can determine whether or not treatment should proceed is the ultimate prognosis of the patient, unless the patient has expressed his views in advance (Dimond, 2005).

---

**Box 12.3 Case study 2: capacity**

Frank is an 82-year-old man who underwent major surgery 6 days ago. Initially, his post-operative recovery was uneventful but after 3 days he began to deteriorate. He has become very weak and needs increasing drug dosages to maintain his cardiorespiratory function and to control his pain and it is likely that he will not survive. His son has requested that should Frank suffer a cardiac arrest that resuscitation be withheld as he feels Frank would not wish to be kept alive in such circumstances.

What is the position of healthcare professionals in these circumstances?

---

All patients who have mental capacity have the right to decide what happens to their body, and their autonomous choices must be consulted whenever possible as the basis of any decision. Patients have capacity to make a decision if they have the capacity to understand the material information, to make a judgement about the information in light of their values, to intend a certain outcome and to communicate freely their wishes to care givers (Beauchamp & Childress, 2001).

There are a number of issues here that the healthcare professional needs to consider.

1 Was Tilly (Case study 3, Box 12.4) mentally competent when she stated that she would not wish to be resuscitated?

If she was, then her autonomous decision should be respected and resuscitation should be withheld.

2 Was Tilly's decision not to be resuscitated as a result of her depression?

If it was, then the decision would be considered to be made during a period of incompetence and she should therefore be treated according to her best interests should she suffer a cardiac arrest.

---

**Box 12.4 Case study 3: autonomy and competence**

Tilly is an 85-year-old lady who underwent major surgery 6 days ago. She has had a fairly uneventful post-operative recovery but today she has developed severe hypotension, which is worsening despite increasing interventions. Her doctor and the nurses caring for her are becoming very concerned about her condition. Her family are informed of the potential seriousness of the situation.

Tilly lived independently in her own home with aid from social services prior to surgery and it is felt, should she recover, she would be very likely to return to the reasonable quality of life she had previously experienced. She does, however, suffer from arthritis, which affects her mobility, her eyesight and hearing are failing and she has become very depressed as the result of the death of her husband 11 months ago.

Her son and daughter have now requested that should she suffer a cardiac arrest that resuscitation is withheld as Tilly had expressed on several occasions that she would not wish to be resuscitated.

What is the position of healthcare professionals in these circumstances?

---

3 Is resuscitation futile in this case?

If it is considered futile, there is no legal obligation to resuscitate.

4 Would Tilly have a chance of a reasonable prognosis if resuscitation were to be instigated?

If so, resuscitation is not considered futile and should therefore be carried out.

Where there is any doubt, healthcare professionals should always err on the side of saving life. Healthcare professionals should take into account relatives wishes during any decision-making process but in deciding whether or not to resuscitate a patient, these views should not be the only consideration (Dimond, 2005).

---

**Box 12.5 Case study 4: autonomy and competence**

Celia, is a 67-year-old lady who, for most of her life, generally enjoyed good health but was diagnosed with multiple sclerosis 8 months previously. The disease has not yet debilitated her seriously. Four days ago, she underwent major surgery for a bowel obstruction and prior to going for surgery, she produced an advance directive, signed by her and witnessed by her friend, stating that should she suffer a cardiac arrest she does not wish to be resuscitated. She has now collapsed following ventricular fibrillation and requires immediate resuscitation if her life is to be saved.

What is the position of healthcare professionals in these circumstances?

---

In acute care settings, there are often circumstances when the hitherto patient with capacity has become incapacitated and is temporarily unable, or no longer able, to make an autonomous choice. In this situation, decisions that have been made while the patient had capacity should be respected and Celia (Case study 4, Box 12.5) should not be resuscitated.

The legal and moral duty of care that is owed to vulnerable clients by those entrusted with their care is of vital importance and must not be overlooked (Fletcher & Buka, 1999).

## THE MENTAL CAPACITY ACT 2005

The Mental Capacity Act 2005 for England and Wales gained Royal Assent on 7 April 2007, and was implemented in stages during 2007. The purpose of the Act is to provide a legal framework to protect vulnerable people who may be assessed as being unable to make informed decisions regarding their own life and choices. The Act provides guidance on the decision-making process where decisions are being made on behalf of those who lack capacity; for example, people with a dementia, learning disability, mental illness or brain injury. The Act also provides guidance for individuals who wish to make provision for their future when they may become sufficiently incapacitated to be able to make rational decisions for themselves. Anyone caring for, or working with, a person who lacks capacity to consent must consult the Act and the corresponding Code of Practice when making any decisions on behalf of someone else, whether these decisions are life-saving or just about everyday matters. The Act clearly outlines who can take these decisions on behalf of another person, identifies the situations where this can take place, and how this works in practice.

The Act sets out some guiding value-based principles that underpin the implementation of the Act itself. There are five statutory principles within the Act that encourage choice and independence. These principles advocate maximising the opportunity for people to be enabled to make their own decisions wherever possible. The five key principles are as follows.

1. A presumption of capacity – every adult has the right to make his or her decisions and must be assumed to have capacity to do so unless it is proved otherwise;
2. The right for individuals to be supported to make their own decisions – people must be given all appropriate help before anyone concludes that they cannot make their own decisions;
3. That individuals must retain the right to make what might be seen as eccentric or unwise decisions;
4. Best interests – anything done for or on behalf of people without capacity must be in their best interests; and
5. Least restrictive intervention – anything done for or on behalf of people without capacity should be the least restrictive of their basic rights and freedoms.

The Act is divided into three parts:

Part 1  Persons who lack capacity,
Part 2  The Court of Protection and the Public Guardian,
Part 3  Miscellaneous and general.

### Capacity to consent
The Act identifies a single test, the 'decision specific' test, which is to be used to determine whether a person lacks capacity. No

longer can this decision be made upon the condition or illness that someone has, or even what decisions they have made so far in life. If the decisions being made are based on medical interventions or treatments then the assessment test is carried out by the specialist medical practitioners who are recommending the treatment. Reasons for bringing capacity into question, proposed treatments, assessments and their results should all be fully documented and recorded in all medical and nursing notes.

An individual will be deemed to be lacking capacity if at the point when the decision needs to be made, they fail to:

- understand the information relevant to the decision,
- retain the information relevant to the decision,
- use or weigh the information, or
- communicate the decision (by any means).

If this is the case then they will be deemed as lacking capacity to consent. If an individual fails to meet one or more of the above sections then the whole test is rendered 'failed' (Department for Constitutional Affairs, 2005).

### Mental Capacity Act: Code of Practice

Whereas the Act provides a Code of Practice it is not law that all individuals adhere to the guidelines set within in it; however, the Code of Practice clearly identifies categories of people who have a legal requirement to 'have a regard' for the Code and when making decisions for clients who lack capacity they must adhere to the guidelines of the Code. Nursing staff caring for people who lack capacity fall into this category. All people within the identified categories must be able to state how they have had and shown regard for the Code and implemented its guidelines.

If any person who does not have a legal requirement to 'have regard' for the Code, such as carers, family or friends, does not follow guidelines in their decision-making and divert from the guidance, then they will be expected to justify why they departed from the guidelines.

The Mental Capacity Act and its Code of Practice (2005) are widely available for all to use. As with all legislation and changes in practice it is every healthcare professional's responsibility to ensure that they are familiar with the Act's guidelines and changes in practice (Department for Constitutional Affairs, 2005).

To illustrate how the Mental Capacity Act affects the incapacitated person and their carers, consider the following case studies (Boxes 12.6 and 12.7).

---

**Box 12.6 Case study 5: Mental Capacity Act and incapacity**

Sally is an 82-year-old lady who has been diagnosed with dementia. When she was diagnosed she told her daughter that she wanted her to help her with things that she had started to find difficult, such as her financial affairs, shopping, planning and arranging appointments. Sally continued to allow her daughter to help her but always maintained that she wanted to make her own decisions and did so with no difficulties. Sally has agreed with her daughter that under the new Mental Capacity Act her daughter will have Lasting Power of Attorney (LPA). When/if the time comes that Sally is assessed as not having capacity to consent or make decisions for herself then this LPA will enable her daughter to make decisions on behalf of Sally.

Sally (donor) will need to nominate her daughter (attorney) and register the LPA with the Office of the Public Guardian (OPG), all regulations and procedures are set out in the Code of Practice.

*A year after the LPA had been registered,* a salesman from a window company called on Sally while she was alone at home. She agreed to have all her windows replaced and signed a cheque for £2000 as a deposit. She already has UPVc windows and certainly did not need replacement windows or doors. Her daughter was not aware of the problem until the cheque was cashed. Fortunately, the company agreed to cancel the work but insisted that

*Continued*

---

they retained the deposit as the windows had already been made.

Sally had no recollection of the caller and since this incident there have been several incidents where Sally has been extremely financially vulnerable. She has handed over too much money at tills, and she has given neighbours large sums of money for shopping. Fortunately, they have been honest and advised Sally's daughter of the incidents.

Sally's daughter is extremely worried about her mother's ability to make informed financial decisions and now needs to have greater input into the control of Sally's financial affairs, she will now need to fully utilise the powers that she has under the LPA (see Code of Practice). It is vitally important that although Sally's daughter will now control her financial affairs, Sally will continue to be enabled and encouraged to make her own decisions about other aspects of her life wherever possible.

---

**Box 12.7 Case study 6: Mental Capacity Act and capacity**

Albert is 79 years old and has suffered with dementia for several years. Albert is currently on an acute admission ward in a psychiatric hospital. Until recently, Albert has been able to express his needs and has, with assistance, been able to make his own decisions about his care and treatment. More recently, the symptoms of his dementia have worsened and he has not been able to fully understand the detail of information that the nurses and doctors are giving him. Albert's short-term memory is extremely poor, his concentration is poor and he is unable to communicate verbally. He has become extremely aggressive and, at times, violent. Albert has been assessed as being unable to give informed consent. Albert has no known next of kin; he was never married, had no children and his brother, his only known relative, died a few months ago.

Albert is now unable to live alone in his bungalow and the multi disciplinary team agree that Albert would be best cared for within a Registered Nursing Home on a permanent basis. Given that Albert has no known next of kin or appointed person who is dealing with his affairs, under the Mental Capacity Act the team will need to refer his case to the Independent Mental Capacity Advocate (IMCA).

The IMCA will:

- be independent of the person making the decision,
- provide support for the person who lacks capacity,
- represent the person without capacity in discussions to work out whether the proposed decision is in the person's best interests,
- provide information to help work out what is in the person's best interests,
- raise questions or challenge decisions that appear not to be in the best interests of the person.

## THE ETHICS OF WITHDRAWAL OF ACTIVE TREATMENT

Difficulties may arise in the acute care setting when caring for patients at the end of their lives, who are unable to make decisions about continuation of treatment. Ethical dilemmas arise when there is a perceived conflicting duty to the patient, such as a conflict between the duty to preserve life and a duty to act in the patient's best interests, or when an ethical principle such as respect for autonomy conflicts with the duty not to harm.

Healthcare professionals have no obligation to offer treatments or procedures that do not benefit patients. Futile treatments are ill-advised because they often increase a patient's pain and discomfort in the last days and weeks of life, and because they can expend finite medical resources (Jecker, 2000).

The principle of beneficence is a moral obligation to act to benefit others or to act in the best interests of others. In healthcare, this may seem obvious as an obligation but there is a risk that we can begin to believe we know what is best for them. In our wish to do good for the patient we can override their autonomy and step beyond the boundary of beneficence into paternalism; that is, the overriding of one person's preferences by another person and possibly inflicting harm.

The ethical principle of non-maleficence – the obligation not to inflict harm intentionally – is important here. Many treatments and procedures in healthcare cause harmful side effects but the interventions save or improve quality of life overall. However, on occasion, the patient's quality of life is so poor or the intervention would prove so burdensome that it is more appropriate to withhold or withdraw it, as the balance of harm over benefit is too great. The major considerations in end-of-life decision-making are the degree of harm being caused by the interventions, whether that harm outweighs any benefits and, indeed, whether death would be a harm in the circumstances.

It is justifiable to discontinue life-sustaining treatments if:

- the patient has the ability to make decisions, fully understands the consequences of their decision and states that they no longer want a treatment,
- the treatment no longer offers benefit to the patient.

(Braddock, 1999)

Although many healthcare professionals feel that it is more acceptable not to start a treatment than to withdraw it, there is actually no ethical distinction between withholding and withdrawing treatment (Braddock, 1999).

A number of ethical doctrines are relevant when considering the withdrawal of treatment and end-of-life decisions.

### Sanctity of life doctrine

According to this doctrine, all human life has worth and therefore it is wrong to end a person's life, directly or indirectly, however poor the quality of that life. In healthcare this would mean preserving life at all costs but clearly, quality of life is hugely important to the majority of people. It is, however, very difficult to objectively assess the quality of a patient's life when you are not living that life. There may though, be circumstances where a patient's quality of life is deemed so poor, it is considered to be a life not worth living and therefore should not be maintained even if it is possible to do so.

### Acts and omissions doctrine

This doctrine highlights the distinction between killing and letting die. There is a moral distinction between taking action to bring about a person's death and refraining from an action that may save or preserve a person's life. For example, it is morally wrong to push someone who cannot swim into deep water; however, there is no moral duty to dive into a river to save someone who is drowning. In the context of healthcare, this would mean it is wrong to give a lethal injection to end a patient's life but treatments that could sustain life can be withdrawn when they are no longer of benefit and therefore it is not in the best interests of the patient to continue. Withholding and withdrawing treatment are both considered omissions to act.

### Doctrine of double effect

This doctrine asserts that there is a moral distinction between carrying out an action to bring about a person's death and carrying out an action that will provide some benefit but as a result the death of the person is a foreseen but unintended consequence. For example, giving high dosages of drugs to relieve pain (beneficial action) which will, however, shorten life (unintended consequence). The intention is to relieve pain but the death of the person is unintended although foreseeable.

## PALLIATIVE CARE IN THE ACUTE SETTING

Palliative care is directed primarily at providing symptom and pain management to patients who are terminally ill and further interventions are inappropriate. The aim of palliative care is not curative but to provide comfort and the highest possible quality of life for as long as life remains, dictated by the concepts of beneficence and justice. The focus is not on death but on ensuring the life that remains is as comfortable as possible.

In considering the appropriateness of palliative care, sanctity versus quality of life issues need to be taken into account. The acts and omissions doctrine and the doctrine of double effect can be very useful in aiding the healthcare deliverer in determining treatment and care options.

For example, the question of whether a patient's life is not worth living because his/her quality of life is so poor as determined by the patient and/or significant others together with the healthcare team can aid the decision whether to withhold or withdraw particular treatments. Omitting to act is justifiable if the action is of no benefit to the patient. Increasing drug dosages to maintain a pain-free state for the patient is acceptable even if that action will bring about death more swiftly because death is the unintended consequence of the beneficent act of killing pain.

**Pain control**

Pain is one of the most common symptoms at the end of life in acute care areas. It is also one of the most unacceptable symptoms in modern healthcare in view of the myriad drugs and treatments that are available for its alleviation. The doctrine of double effect is important here, together with the principle of beneficence. The question that arises here is whether death (a harm in the circumstance) is an acceptable outcome. If the answer is that life is too burdensome for the patient, then it could be considered a life not worth living and death would not be a harm but indeed a release from pain and therefore burden. The best person to determine the answer to this question is the patient. Pain reduces quality of life, so if pain is alleviated, the burden to the patient is reduced and quality of life improves even if that life is shorter as a result of the treatments given.

SUMMARY

- Ethical theories, principles and doctrines should be considered in decision-making processes at the end of life as they will provide a useful framework.
- DNAR orders should only be used in specific circumstances and where possible following discussion and agreement with the patient (respect for autonomy).
- Advance directives should be made by individuals who have mental capacity and the provisions within it will negate legal proceedings if the doctor believes the content to be the true wishes of the patient.

- Treatment can be withdrawn or withheld if it is deemed to be futile or if harm caused by the intervention outweighs the benefits (non-maleficence).
- It is ethically justifiable to administer treatments that alleviate unacceptable symptoms even though they will inevitably shorten life.

## REFERENCES

Beauchamp, TL & Childress, JF (2001) *Principles of Biomedical Ethics*, 5th edn. Oxford University Press, Oxford

Bosek, MS & Savage, TA (2007) *The Ethical Component of Nursing Education: Integrating Ethics into Clinical Experience*. Lippincott Williams and Wilkins, London

Bowker, L & Stewart, K (1999) Predicting unsuccessful cardiopulmonary resuscitation (CPR): a comparison of three morbidity scores. *Resuscitation* **40**, 89–95

Braddock, CH (1999) *Termination of Life-Sustaining Treatment*. http://dets.washington.edu/bioethx/topics/termlife.html (accessed 27 April 2007)

Department for Constitutional Affairs (2005) *Mental Capacity Act: Code of Practice*. The Stationery Office, London [issued by the Lord Chancellor on 23 April 2007 in accordance with sections 42 and 43 of the Act]

Dimond, B (2005) *Legal Aspects of Nursing*, 4th edn. Pearson Longman, Harlow

Ewanchuck, M & Brindley, PG (2006) *Ethics Review: Perioperative Do-not-Resuscitate Orders – Doing 'Nothing' When Something Can be Done*. www.ccforum.com (accessed 15 April 2007)

Fletcher, L & Buka, P (1999) *A Legal Framework for Caring: an Introduction to Law and Ethics in Heath Care*. Macmillan, London

Jecker, NS (2000) *Futility*. http://depts.washington.edu/bioethx/topics/futil.html (accessed 27 April 2007)

Nursing and Midwifery Council (2008) *Code of Professional Conduct*. Nursing and Midwifery Council, London

Wacker Guido, G (2006) *Legal and Ethical Issues in Nursing*, 4th edn. Pearson Prentice Hall, New Jersey

**Mental Capacity Act websites**
www.dca.gov.uk/menincap/legis.htm
www.opsi.gov.uk/acts/acts2005/20050009.htm

# Index